Neonatal Resuscitation with Placental Circulation Intact

Neonatal Resuscitation with Placental Circulation Intact

Editors

Simone Pratesi
David Hutchon
Anup Katheria

MDPI • Basel • Beijing • Wuhan • Barcelona • Belgrade • Manchester • Tokyo • Cluj • Tianjin

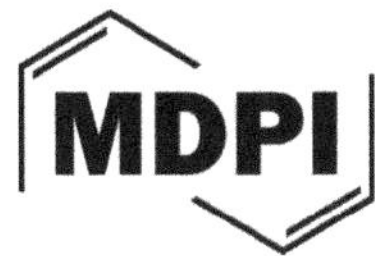

Editors

Simone Pratesi	David Hutchon	Anup Katheria
Careggi University Hospital	Darlington Memorial	Neonatal Research Institute
Florence	Hospital	and NICU follow-up Clinic at
Italy	Darlington	Sharp Mary Birch Hospital
	United Kingdom	University of California
		San Diego
		United States

Editorial Office
MDPI
St. Alban-Anlage 66
4052 Basel, Switzerland

This is a reprint of articles from the Special Issue published online in the open access journal *Children* (ISSN 2227-9067) (available at: www.mdpi.com/journal/children/special_issues/Neonatal_Resuscitation_with_Placental_Circulation_Intact).

For citation purposes, cite each article independently as indicated on the article page online and as indicated below:

LastName, A.A.; LastName, B.B.; LastName, C.C. Article Title. *Journal Name* **Year**, *Volume Number*, Page Range.

ISBN 978-3-0365-7935-1 (Hbk)
ISBN 978-3-0365-7934-4 (PDF)

Cover image courtesy of Satyan Lakshminrusimha

Contents

About the Editors

Simone Pratesi

Simone Pratesi is an Associate Professor of Pediatrics at Florence University, and received their Ph.D. in Perinatology at Roma La Sapienza University. Pratesi has also been a teacher in neonatal resuscitation for the Italian Society of Neonatology since 2003, and a trainer in high-fidelity simulation for the Italian Society of Neonatology since 2014. Their main clinical and research interests and experience include neonatal jaundice, conventional and fiberoptic phototherapy of neonatal jaundice, transcutaneous measurement of bilirubin, non-invasive monitoring of neonatal cerebral oxygenation and hemodynamics with near-infrared spectroscopy, transitional circulation, patent ductus arteriosus, neonatal resuscitation, delayed cord clamping, neonatal resuscitation with an intact cord, and pediatric cardiology and echocardiography.

David Hutchon

David J R Hutchon is an Emeritus Consultant Obstetrician at the Darlington Memorial Hospital after 35 years of clinical practice. He has spent the last 10 years studying and teaching about the circulatory changes which occur at birth and the importance of residual placental circulation. He has published more than 20 papers on the subject and is an Editorial Board Member of the *Maternal Health, Neonatology and Perinatology* journal. He led the team whose research resulted in the production of the first mobile neonatal resuscitation trolley, now being used in a number of units in the UK, Europe and the USA.

Anup Katheria

Dr. Anup Katheria is an Associate Professor of Pediatrics and the Director of the Neonatal Research Institute and NICU follow-up clinic at Sharp Mary Birch Hospital for Women & Newborns. His research interests include functional echocardiography, point-of-care ultrasound, and conducting clinical trials. He is currently conducting several large multicenter trials: 1. comparing cord milking to early cord clamping in term non-vigorous infants; 2. comparing delayed cord clamping to umbilical cord milking in preterm infants; 3. Comparing empiric antibiotic therapy to placebo in extremely low-birthweight infants; 4 comparing early CPAP to early minimal invasive surfactant administration (LISA); 5. evaluating the use of cromolyn therapy to reduce BPD; and 6. comparing the effectiveness of nasal high-flow cannula to CPAP. Dr. Katheria earned his BS in Biology from the University of California, Los Angeles and his MD from Drexel University College of Medicine. He completed his pediatric residency at Children's Hospital of Orange County, and his Neonatal-Perinatal Fellowship at the University of California, San Diego.

Preface to "Neonatal Resuscitation with Placental Circulation Intact"

Neonatal transitional physiology should include a delay in cord clamping until after the newborn is breathing: this is easy to perform in a healthy term newborn, but not in a sick or preterm newborn. A delayed cord clamping of 30 seconds reduces the hospital mortality of preterm newborns. Very limited data are available on delayed cord clamping in term newborns who require neonatal resuscitation at birth. Resuscitation with an intact cord is feasible and safe, both in term and preterm newborns, and could be the best way to stabilize a newborn in the delivery room. Immediate cord clamping still represents the standard care in very preterm and sick newborns worldwide. To promote a different, more physiological approach to newborns in need of assistance at birth, neonatologists should move close to the delivering mother to evaluate the tone, heart rate, and breathing efforts of the newborn, and at least start the initial steps of stabilization (above all, breathing tactile stimulation) before the cord is clamped. Recent studies have demonstrated that resuscitating a newborn with an intact cord is safely feasible, both with and without the use of special equipment and a movable trolley. However, these special devices still need technological improvements and are too expensive to permit the rapid spread of this approach in delivery room care protocols. The goal of this research topic is to promote the spread of a new way of resuscitating newborns in the delivery room, which comprises performing exactly the same neonatal resuscitation procedures (according to the 2020 neonatal resuscitation guidelines) in a different landscape, that is, at the mother's side with an intact cord. Authors have been invited to contribute to this Special Issue with original research or clinical trial articles, study protocols, brief research, case report articles, and technology and code articles, addressing themes such as the following:

1) Delayed cord clamping, which is longer than 1 minute after the newborn breathes, in preterm babies;

2) Neonatal resuscitation/assistance with an intact cord in preterm newborns;

3) Neonatal resuscitation with an intact cord in asphyxiated term newborns;

4) Neonatal resuscitation with an intact cord in congenital fetal anomalies (hydrops fetalis, diaphragmatic hernia, etc.);

5) Technological advances (trolley, heating system, ventilation system, etc.) to promote neonatal assistance with an intact cord;

6) High-fidelity simulation to promote multiprofessional neonatal assistance with an intact cord;

7) Physiological (hemodynamic and respiratory) neonatal adaptation during an intact cord transition (both animal and human studies).

I am really grateful to all authors for their valuable work, and to David Hutchon and Anup Katheria for their expert assistance as co-Editors of this Special Issue of *Children*. Special thanks to Satyan Lakshminrusimha for making the cover figure for the reprint.

Simone Pratesi, David Hutchon, and Anup Katheria

Editors

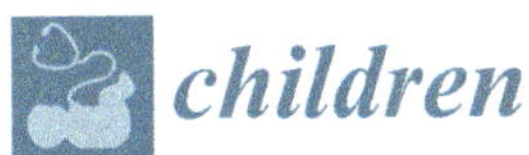

Editorial

How to Provide Motherside Neonatal Resuscitation with Intact Placental Circulation?

David Hutchon [1], Simone Pratesi [2,*] and Anup Katheria [3]

1 Emeritus Consultant Obstetrician, Memorial Hospital, Darlington DL3 6HX, UK; djrhutchon@hotmail.co.uk
2 Neonatology Unit, Careggi University Hospital, 50134 Florence, Italy
3 Neonatal Research Institute Sharp Mary Birch Hospital for Women & Newborns, San Diego, CA 92123, USA; Anup.Katheria@sharp.com
* Correspondence: simone.pratesi@unifi.it

Citation: Hutchon, D.; Pratesi, S.; Katheria, A. How to Provide Motherside Neonatal Resuscitation with Intact Placental Circulation?. *Children* **2021**, *8*, 291. https://doi.org/10.3390/children8040291

Received: 22 March 2021
Accepted: 6 April 2021
Published: 8 April 2021

Publisher's Note: MDPI stays neutral with regard to jurisdictional claims in published maps and institutional affiliations.

Immediate clamping and cutting of the umbilical cord have been associated with death and/or neurodisability [1–5]. Given the harm from immediate cord clamping it would seem logical that all infants should receive delayed cord clamping, but evidence for delayed cord clamping when resuscitation is required is limited. One approach would be to perform resuscitation while the cord is still intact. Several studies have demonstrated improvements in physiological outcomes, such as higher Apgar scores or oxygen levels in the first few minutes of birth with resuscitation with an intact cord compared to early cord clamping [6–11]. Another challenge, however, is implementation of this practice. While some groups have reported this practice to be relatively straightforward [11–16], others have struggled with its implementation [17]. Resuscitation equipment and procedures need to be acceptable to clinicians and parents for use outside a research environment [17–19]. Modifications of the equipment and increased co-operation between obstetric and neonatal teams are required. Practice and training are prerequisites to ensuring that resuscitation at the side of the mother with an intact placental circulation provides the same standard of care for the neonate and permit the obstetrical team to provide unhindered care for the mother. The care must meet International Liaison Committee on Resuscitation (ILCOR) [20] and other neonatal and obstetric standards, and adapt as new evidence emerges. For example, the guidance for the application of mask positive pressure ventilation in the poorly breathing neonate [21] may need to be reviewed in the light of evidence showing that mask application may actually precipitate apnoea and bradycardia [22]. Many preterm and some apparently asphyxiated term neonates will only require time to stabilise transition with an intact placental circulation while remaining on the resuscitation equipment. International guidelines for neonatal resuscitation suggest to delay cord clamping at birth for at least 30 s in preterm newborns whenever feasible, but there are no guidelines for neonatal providers [20]. This review aims to provide guidance for how neonatal providers can support placental transfusion for all infants, particularly the extremely preterm infant.

There are several resuscitation trolleys that are available for research use. Two are commercially available in Europe (CONCORD and LifeStart Trolley) and others are under research protocols (INSPIRE and NOOMA). No matter which is used, all should have some of the basic features as shown in Table 1.

1. Equipment for Neonatal Resuscitation with Placental Circulation Intact

Neonatal resuscitation equipment needs to be designed to allow for routine resuscitation with an intact placental circulation. At the same time the obstetric team needs to have access to provide any necessary care to for the mother. A stable platform which can be brought right up to the mother close enough for an intact cord may require modification and integration with the various designs of birthing tables. The practice of delayed clamping with resuscitation remains mostly as part of research protocols. This may be because concerns remain about the need for immediate resuscitation, or situations where there may be an imminent delivery without adequate time to setup equipment or space for extra personnel. Currently, two specially designed neonatal resuscitation trollies are available for resuscitation with an intact cord. While resuscitation with an intact cord can be achieved with standard equipment some of the above previously stated challenges may continue [23,24].

Table 1. Basic features to be assured in motherside neonatal resuscitation.

1.   A stable flat, soft, but firm surface on which to place safely the neonate during resuscitation.
2.   Warming equipment to prevent hypothermia. Preterm babies placed in a polythene bag while under the radiant heater are usually able to maintain their body temperature.
3.   Good lighting
4.   All the equipment to provide positive pressure ventilation with positive end-expiratory pressure (PEEP) immediately and easily available. The neonatologist can personally adjust the settings and oxygen levels if necessary. Suction is available. Other accessory equipment possibly available in store compartments.
5.   Monitoring equipment available or accessible on or immediately near the trolley.
6.   Easy access to the trolley allowing a team to provide resuscitation.

2. Design Features Required to Meet All Criteria for Current Standard Resuscitation

The precise requirements will vary between the two main modes of birth, assisted vaginal birth and caesarean section. While neonates born naturally sometimes need resuscitation this is infrequent and the equipment and procedure can be more readily dealt with. The equipment at assisted births needs specific requirements. A major consideration at caesarean section is maintaining the integrity of the sterile field. This needs the neonatal resuscitation team to be part of the sterile field. Provided nothing passes from the neonatal team to the obstetric team after the neonate is delivered, some compromise to the equipment used by the neonatal team may be acceptable.

2.1. Platform

The surface of the platform should be flat to provide an optimal position for an open airway ("sniffing position"). It should be at a height which allows the neonatal team to provide the care necessary. The surface should be soft and firm. It must be stable so that the neonate can be placed on the surface without any risk of the platform moving or risk of the neonate falling off the platform. The platform should be of a sufficient size to accommodate also large term neonates and must be capable of getting as close as possible to the vaginal introitus or caesarean incision, as the cord must not be under tension for it to remain functional. In case of caesarean section, it can be covered with sterile drapes as is normal for the Mayo table.

2.2. Platform Position and Access by Neonatal Team

With a specialized resuscitation trolley, three sides of the trolley can be easily accessed by a member of the resuscitation team. Figure 1 shows four possible positions for the platform during caesarean section.

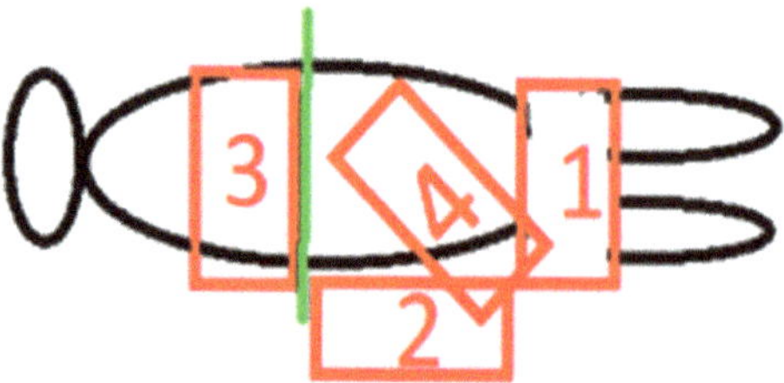

Figure 1. Possible positions for the platform during caesarean section.

Position 1, over the mother's thighs seems the most straightforward position. Provided the platform is relatively thin, the surface can be virtually at the level of the uterus/placenta. It needs to be supported and not resting on the mother's thighs. Only one person can have ready access to the neonate.

Position 2, at the side of the operating table is the normal position for the operating obstetrician, so this position requires the obstetrician to move away during the resuscitation. This position gives access for two or possibly three people around the resuscitation platform. The platform can be lowered to be significantly below the level of the placenta provided there is sufficient cord length. The surgical assistant remains to deal with the surgical wound and delivery of the placenta if necessary. Rarely will there be any significant problem during the few minutes after a birth. After about three minutes or earlier delivery of the placenta there is no physiological advantage for the resuscitation procedure to remain at the side of the mother.

Position 3 is likely to place the neonate significantly above the placental level and may also require the obstetrician to move slightly if there is more than one person providing resuscitation. A sterile screen can be used to separate off the surgical field immediately after delivery of the baby. It is close to the face of the mother, who potentially could see, speak to and touch her baby.

Position 4 is similar to position 1 but probably permit to manage newborn with a shorter cord. This position gives access for two people around the resuscitation platform but requires the obstetrician to move apart during the resuscitation.

In all four positions there needs to be an independent support for the platform which provides sufficient stability as well as mobility to get into position immediately after the birth and away again three to five minutes later. It needs to be able to accommodate height differences especially if it is also used at assisted vaginal birth. If the trolley is customised for caesarean birth only then the range of height adjustment is significantly reduced. The height of the operating table could be adjusted to meet the requirements of the resuscitation platform.

The resuscitation platform has significantly different height requirements for caesarean section as for assisted vaginal birth. Enterprising design is required to make the specialized equipment provide the same standards as routine resuscitation beds. At assisted vaginal birth it is inevitable that the platform to place the baby will be lower than the height of the standard resuscitation equipment. Raising the birthing table may help to reduce this compromise. The mother's legs, in the lithotomy poles may also limit access and require the obstetrician to move away for a short time to allow the neonatal team access.

A specialized trolley which provides the facility for resuscitation with intact placental circulation at both caesarean births and assisted vaginal births may compromise the facility for both modes of birth, and separate designs may be preferable. Most assisted vaginal births do not take place in the caesarean room, so equipment customised for an assisted vaginal birth can remain in the labour ward delivery room, while equipment customised for caesarean births can remain in the operating room.

The cost of the equipment is obviously a serious consideration, but, given the enormous cost of the lifelong care of an individual with hypoxic birth injury [9], and the cost and effort of trying to mitigate any damage of hypoxic ischaemia at birth [25], even preventing a small proportion of injuries with resuscitation during an intact placental circulation could pay for the equipment many times over [9,25,26].

2.3. Heating and Prevention of Hypothermia

A standard resuscitation bed is equipped by an overhead radiant heater. The resuscitation platform of the trolley can also be warmed if the heater is switched on for a short time before the equipment is required, however this may be ineffective compared to radiant heat. The preterm neonate's body is enclosed in polythene, a cap is placed on the neonatal head and warmed towels placed around its body. Chemical heating mattresses can be used to provide additional heating. Some types of mattress seem to be efficacious in maintaining normothermia (36.5–37.5 °C) even without an overhead radiant heater, but body temperature should be accurately checked in the delivery room. Instead, if such mattresses are used in combination with a radiant heater, hyperthermia (>38 °C) should be checked and avoided. The ambient temperature of the delivery room (23–25 °C, and >25° for newborns less than 28 wks) is important to reduce the risk of hypothermia even with all the above measures. The ambient temperature should be checked in the delivery room and promptly increased while assisting a very preterm delivery.

Providing the equipment for warming during these first few minutes after birth at motherside is a significant challenge. The possibility of the traditional radiant heater is limited at both caesarean section and vaginal births due to limited access immediately above the resuscitation platform. A temporary radiant heater could be used in positions 1 and 3, possibly attached to the operating light and only turned on immediately before the birth.

A warming mattress is available on one of the commercially available trollies, but, for preterm neonates, it may not be sufficient and supplementary chemical heating units have been effectively used. The ambient temperature of the air is extremely important and a warm theatre temperature is required for the safety of these neonates.

The use of a sterile polythene bag, covering also the head of the infant, presents no additional problem at caesarean section.

2.4. Equipment

Newborns who do not start breathing efficaciously after proper stimulation should be supported by nCPAP or positive pressure ventilation (PPV) within 1 min of life. In high-resource settings the initial provision of PPV is with a T-piece ventilator providing PEEP, (positive end expiratory pressure) with carefully controlled PIP (peak inspiratory pressure). A number of items of equipment are commercially available which provide PEEP and PIP with visible gauges showing the set pressure levels [27]. A suction device and warmed and humidified gas for the inspired gas is ideal. The user, or another member of the resuscitation team, controls the pressure levels during resuscitation. Resuscitation with PPV is normally started with air in term newborns and between 21% and 30% of oxygen in preterm newborns, then oxygen requirement is adjusted on newborn's saturation values, so an increased concentration of oxygen needs to be available via a blender. Again, oxygen concentration is displayed and controlled by the clinician or another member of the resuscitation team if necessary.

The equipment to provide ventilation and suction can be remote or within the structure supporting the platform. International guidelines for neonatal resuscitation do not recommend routine oral, nasal, or oropharyngeal suctioning of the newborn at birth [20], and equipment could be useful only in case of suspected airway obstruction during positive pressure ventilation. Since some supporting framework is essential for all four positions, it seems logical, if possible, to include the ventilation equipment within the framework. If the equipment is remote then adjustment and monitoring of the pressure, flow and oxygen level by the neonatologist providing PPV is not feasible and requires a second person taking instructions. It also requires tubing from the remote equipment to the resuscitation platform which has an additional risk of compromising the sterile field. Providing all the equipment within the standard roomside resuscitation trolley into the motherside trolley is a considerable design challenge. Standard resuscitation equipment has centralised gas supply of air and oxygen and suction with an emergency backup of cylinders of air and oxygen. The gas supply for the ventilatory equipment is also a challenge. Tubing can be brought from standard outlets but these are cumbersome and limit the mobility of the trolley. They present a hazard within the theatre. Small cylinders can also be fitted but these are inevitably heavy and have a very limited supply.

2.5. Monitoring

Increasingly, more sophisticated monitoring is being used routinely. The minimal requirement is for heart rate and lung air entry via a stethoscope and also pulse oximetry. Electronic equipment for monitoring the neonatal parameters such as heart rate and oxygen saturation at birth are rapidly developing. In terms of size, weight, and sterility, none of these should present any difficulty in having them available on a mobile resuscitation trolley, but still they have not. Wireless transmission of signals makes it possible to include the equipment within the caesarean section sterile field if this can be contained within a sterile container.

2.6. Mobility

Roomside neonatal resuscitation trollies are generally stable and mobile enough so that if extended care is required the neonate can be moved to the special care nursery on the trolley. This is provided there is an independent gas supply on the machine. However, a transport incubator is frequently used to move the newborn from delivery room to neonatal intensive care unit.

Motherside neonatal resuscitation trolley is not intended to be used to move the neonate, but being mobile, it must also be capable of having a safe and stable platform for resuscitation of the neonate. Stability normally requires a large base but a large base limits mobility and proximity to the operating table.

3. Conclusions

Although the intervention of early cord clamping has no advantage for the mother or the baby, it is a reality that neonatal resuscitation was introduced while the practice was already established. Current practice and guidelines are based on the premise that there is unrestricted access to the neonate. The World Health Organisation (WHO) suggests that resuscitation with the cord intact is dependent upon the skill of the neonatologist [1]. A change in practice to remove the harmful intervention of early cord clamping in conjunction with neonatal resuscitation will require other changes in practice and the development of equipment that supports resuscitation procedures close to the mother and the obstetric team delivering the neonate. Two customised trollies are available commercially [28–30] but have not been obtained by most units throughout Europe and the USA.

Author Contributions: Conceptualization, D.H. and S.P.; methodology, D.H., S.P. and A.K.; data curation, D.H., S.P. and A.K.; writing—original draft preparation, D.H.; writing—review and editing, S.P. and A.K. All authors have read and agreed to the published version of the manuscript.

Funding: This research received no external funding.

Institutional Review Board Statement: Not applicable.

Informed Consent Statement: Not applicable.

Data Availability Statement: No new data were created or analyzed in this study. Data sharing is not applicable to this article.

Conflicts of Interest: Authors declare that they have no conflict of interest to report.

References

1. Mercer, J.S.; Vohr, B.R.; McGrath, M.M.; Padbury, J.F.; Wallach, M.; Oh, W. Delayed Cord Clamping in Very Preterm Infants Reduces the Incidence of Intraventricular Hemorrhage and Late-Onset Sepsis: A Randomized, Controlled Trial. *Pediatrics* **2006**, *117*, 1235–1242. [CrossRef]
2. Fogarty, M.; Osborn, D.A.; Askie, L.; Seidler, A.L.; Hunter, K.; Lui, K.; Simes, J.; Tarnow-Mordi, W. Delayed vs. early umbilical cord clamping for preterm infants: A systematic review and meta-analysis. *Am. J. Obstet. Gynecol.* **2018**, *218*, 1–18. [CrossRef]
3. Ashish, K.C.; Malqvist, M.; Rana, N.; Ranneberg, L.J.; Andersson, O. Effect of timing of umbilical cord clamping on anemia at 8 and 12 months and later neurodevelopment in late pre-term and term infants; a facility-based, randomized-controlled trial in Nepal. *BMC Pediatr.* **2016**, *16*, 35.
4. Van Rheenen, P. Delayed cord clamping and improved infant outcomes. *BMJ* **2011**, *343*, d7127. [CrossRef]

5. Andersson, O.; Domellöf, M.; Andersson, D.; Hellström-Westas, L. Effect of delayed vs early umbilical cord clamping on iron status and neurodevelopment at age 12 months: A randomized clinical trial. *JAMA Pediatr.* **2014**, *168*, 547–554. [CrossRef]
6. Pratesi, S.; Montano, S.; Ghirardello, S.; Mosca, F.; Boni, L.; Tofani, L.; Dani, C. Placental Circulation Intact Trial (PCI-T)—Resuscitation with the Placental Circulation Intact vs. Cord Milking for Very Preterm Infants: A Feasibility Study. *Front. Pediatr.* **2018**, *6*. [CrossRef]
7. Andersson, O.; Rana, N.; Ewald, U.; Målqvist, M.; Stripple, G.; Basnet, O.; Subedi, K.; Kc, A. Intact cord resuscitation versus early cord clamping in the treatment of depressed newborn infants during the first 10 minutes of birth (Nepcord III)—A randomized clinical trial. *Matern. Health Neonatol. Perinatol.* **2019**, *5*, 1–11. [CrossRef]
8. Polglase, G.R.; Schmölzer, G.M.; Roberts, C.T.; Blank, D.A.; Badurdeen, S.; Crossley, K.J.; Miller, S.L.; Stojanovska, V.; Galinsky, R.; Kluckow, M.; et al. Cardiopulmonary Resuscitation of Asystolic Newborn Lambs Prior to Umbilical Cord Clamping; the Timing of Cord Clamping Matters! *Front. Physiol.* **2020**, *11*, 902. [CrossRef]
9. Martinello, K.; Hart, A.R.; Yap, S.; Mitra, S.; Robertson, N.J. Management and investigation of neonatal encephalopathy: 2017 up-date. *Arch. Dis. Child. Fetal Neonatal Ed.* **2017**, *102*, F346–F358. [CrossRef]
10. Katheria, A.; Poeltler, D.; Durham, J.; Steen, J.; Rich, W.; Arnell, K.; Maldonado, M.; Cousins, L.; Finer, N. Neonatal Resuscitation with an Intact Cord: A Randomized Clinical Trial. *J. Pediatr.* **2016**, *178*, 75–80.e3. [CrossRef]
11. Katheria, A.C.; Brown, M.K.; Faksh, A.; Hassen, K.O.; Rich, W.; Lazarus, D.; Steen, J.; Daneshmand, S.S.; Finer, N.N. Delayed Cord Clamping in Newborns Born at Term at Risk for Resuscitation: A Feasibility Randomized Clinical Trial. *J. Pediatr.* **2017**, *187*, 313–317.e1. [CrossRef] [PubMed]
12. Hutchon, D.; Burleigh, A. Neonatal resuscitation. *AIMS J.* **2013**, *25*, 17.
13. Hutchon, D.J.R. *How to Resuscitate the Neonate with the Cord Intact at Caesarean Section*; British International Congress of Obstetrics and Gynaecology: London, UK, 2007; p. P02.28.
14. Batey, N.; Yoxall, C.W.; Fawke, J.A.; Duley, L.; Dorling, J. Fifteen-minute consultation: Stabilisation of the high-risk newborn infant beside the mother. *Arch. Dis. Child. Educ. Pr. Ed.* **2017**, *102*, 235–238. [CrossRef] [PubMed]
15. Winter, J.; Kattwinkel, J.; Chisholm, C.; Blackman, A.; Wilson, S.; Fairchild, K. Ventilation of Preterm Infants during Delayed Cord Clamping (VentFirst): A Pilot Study of Feasibility and Safety. *Am. J. Perinatol.* **2016**, *34*, 111–116. [CrossRef]
16. Sæther, E.; Gülpen, F.R.-V.; Jensen, C.; Myklebust, T.Å.; Eriksen, B.H. Neonatal transitional support with intact umbilical cord in assisted vaginal deliveries: A quality-improvement cohort study. *BMC Pregnancy Childbirth* **2020**, *20*, 1–14. [CrossRef]
17. Katheria, A.C.; Sorkhi, S.R.; Hassen, K.; Faksh, A.; Ghorishi, Z.; Poeltler, D. Acceptability of Bedside Resuscitation with Intact Umbilical Cord to Clinicians and Patients' Families in the United States. *Front. Pediatr.* **2018**, *6*, 100. [CrossRef]
18. Fulton, C.; Stoll, K.; Thordarson, D. Bedside resuscitation of newborns with an intact umbilical cord: Experiences of midwives from British Columbia. *Midwifery* **2016**, *34*, 42–46. [CrossRef]
19. Thomas, M.R.; Yoxall, C.W.; Weeks, A.D.; Duley, L. Providing newborn resuscitation at the mother's bedside: Assessing the safety, usability and acceptability of a mobile trolley. *BMC Pediatr.* **2014**, *14*, 135. [CrossRef]
20. Aziz, K.; Lee, H.C.; Escobedo, M.B.; Hoover, A.V.; Kamath-Rayne, B.D.; Kapadia, V.S.; Magid, D.J.; Niermeyer, S.; Schmölzer, G.M.; Szyld, E.; et al. Part 5: Neonatal Resuscitation: 2020 American Heart Association Guidelines for Cardiopulmonary Resuscitation and Emergency Cardiovascular Care. *Circulation* **2020**, *142* (Suppl. 2), S524–S550. [CrossRef]
21. Ersdal, H.L.; Mduma, E.; Svensen, E.; Perlman, J.M. Early initiation of basic resuscitation interventions including face mask ventilation may reduce birth asphyxia related mortality in low-income countries: A prospective descriptive observational study. *Resuscitation* **2012**, *83*, 869–873. [CrossRef] [PubMed]
22. Gaertner, V.D.; Rüegger, C.M.; O'Currain, E.; Kamlin, C.O.F.; Hooper, S.B.; Davis, P.G.; Springer, L. Physiological responses to facemask application in newborns immediately after birth. *Arch. Dis. Child. Fetal Neonatal Ed.* **2020**. [CrossRef] [PubMed]
23. Schoonakker, B.D.J.; Dorling, J.; Oddie, S.; Batra, D.; Grace, N.; Duley, L.; Very Preterm Birth Qualitative Collaborative Group. Bedside Resuscitation of Preterm Infants with Cord Intact Is Achievable Using Standard Resuscitaire. In Proceedings of the 54th Annual Meeting, European Society for Paediatric Research, Porto, Portugal, 10–14 October 2013; p. 430, Poster Session "Delivery Room Management #5".
24. Thoresen, M. Supportive Care During Neuroprotective Hypothermia in the Term Newborn: Adverse Effects and Their Prevention. *Clin. Perinatol.* **2008**, *35*, 749–763. [CrossRef]
25. Rennie, J.M. Neonatology. In *Obstetrics by Ten Teachers*, 19th ed.; Bennet, P.N., Kenny, L.C., Eds.; CRC Press: Boca Raton, FL, USA, 2011; p. 286.
26. Hutchon, D.J.R.; Wepster, B. The Estimated Cost of Early Cord Clamping at Birth Within Europe. *Int. J. Childbirth* **2014**, *4*, 250–256. [CrossRef]
27. Bennett, S.; Finer, N.N.; Rich, W.; Vaucher, Y. A comparison of three neonatal resuscitation devices. *Resuscitation* **2005**, *67*, 113–118. [CrossRef] [PubMed]
28. Hutchon, D.; Bettles, N. Motherside care of the term neonate at birth. *Matern. Health Neonatol. Perinatol.* **2016**, *2*, 1–4. [CrossRef]
29. Knol, R.; Brouwer, E.; Vernooij, A.S.N.; Klumper, F.J.C.M.; Dekoninck, P.; Hooper, S.B.; Pas, A.B.T. Clinical aspects of incorporating cord clamping into stabilisation of preterm infants. *Arch. Dis. Child. Fetal Neonatal Ed.* **2018**, *103*, F493–F497. [CrossRef] [PubMed]
30. Concord Neonatal. Available online: https://concordneonatal.com/solution/ (accessed on 8 April 2021).

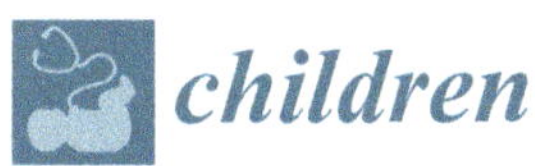 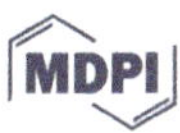

Review

Making the Argument for Intact Cord Resuscitation: A Case Report and Discussion

Judith Mercer [1,2,*], Debra Erickson-Owens [2], Heike Rabe [3], Karen Jefferson [4] and Ola Andersson [5]

1   Neonatal Research Institute, Sharp Mary Birch Hospital for Women and Newborns, San Diego, CA 92123, USA
2   College of Nursing, University of Rhode Island, Kingston, RI 02881, USA; debeo@uri.edu
3   Brighton and Sussex Medical School, University of Sussex, Brighton BN2 5BE, UK; heike.rabe@nhs.net
4   American College of Nurse-Midwives, Silver Spring, MD 20910, USA; kjefferson@acnm.org
5   Department of Clinical Sciences Lund, Paediatrics, Lund University, 221 85 Lund, Sweden; ola.andersson@med.lu.se
*   Correspondence: jsmercer@uri.edu

Abstract: We use a case of intact cord resuscitation to argue for the beneficial effects of an enhanced blood volume from placental transfusion for newborns needing resuscitation. We propose that intact cord resuscitation supports the process of physiologic neonatal transition, especially for many of those newborns appearing moribund. Transfer of the residual blood in the placenta provides the neonate with valuable access to otherwise lost blood volume while changing from placental respiration to breathing air. Our hypothesis is that the enhanced blood flow from placental transfusion initiates mechanical and chemical forces that directly, and indirectly through the vagus nerve, cause vasodilatation in the lung. Pulmonary vascular resistance is thereby reduced and facilitates the important increased entry of blood into the alveolar capillaries before breathing commences. In the presented case, enhanced perfusion to the brain by way of an intact cord likely led to regained consciousness, initiation of breathing, and return of tone and reflexes minutes after birth. Paramount to our hypothesis is the importance of keeping the umbilical cord circulation intact during the first several minutes of life to accommodate physiologic neonatal transition for all newborns and especially for those most compromised infants.

Keywords: intact cord resuscitation; placental transfusion; cord clamping; perfusion; vagus nerve

Citation: Mercer, J.; Erickson-Owens, D.; Rabe, H.; Jefferson, K.; Andersson, O. Making the Argument for Intact Cord Resuscitation: A Case Report and Discussion. *Children* **2022**, *9*, 517. https://doi.org/10.3390/children9040517

Academic Editors: Simone Pratesi, Anup Katheria and David Hutchon

Received: 2 February 2022
Accepted: 24 March 2022
Published: 6 April 2022

Publisher's Note: MDPI stays neutral with regard to jurisdictional claims in published maps and institutional affiliations.

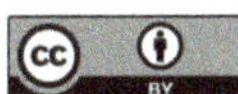

1. Introduction

Around the world, 2.9 million babies die each year at birth from perinatal asphyxia, and a third die within the first day [1]. In many cases, the newborns received immediate or early cord clamping, a non-evidence-based intervention [2]. Waiting to clamp the umbilical cord at birth results in a 30% decreased incidence of death for preterm infants [3–6]. Enhanced blood volume from placental transfusion may be the most important factor that prevents death in these infants [7]. Immediate and early cord clamping can prevent the transfer of essential fetal–neonatal blood volume and interfere with its associated benefits.

Performing resuscitation with an intact cord provides a continuous connection to the placenta, allowing the depressed newborn to have ongoing circulation of fetal–neonatal blood. This action provides cardiovascular stabilization, exchange of oxygen and carbon dioxide, and other support during resuscitation [8,9]. The amount of blood available is significant: for a term newborn, it is about 30% of the fetal–placental blood volume [10]; for a preterm infant, it is up to 50% [11]. Loss of this large blood volume can result in severe hypovolemia and ischemia as the newborn adapts to life without aid from the placenta [12]. Intact umbilical cord milking supports the transfer of some of the blood volume to the newborn quickly, which is beneficial but does not provide for continued connection or respiration [13]. Two recent papers on intact cord resuscitation have reported improvements in infants and newborn animals needing resuscitation. Andersson et al. found higher Apgar scores at 5 and 10 minutes after a three-minute wait for newborns who needed resuscitation compared to those receiving immediate cord clamping [14] and improved neurodevelopment after two years [15]. Polglase reported that in post-asphyxial newborn lambs, a 10-minute delay in cord clamping (after return of systemic circulation) prevented an overshoot of blood pressure (post-asphyxial rebound hypertension). This overshoot was not prevented by either a one-minute wait or immediate cord clamping [16].

Resuscitation with an intact cord is fairly routine in out-of-hospital settings in the US and Canada, but few in-hospital providers have attended such births [17,18]. However, historic references of intact cord resuscitation exist as far back as Aristotle [19]. For those with experience-derived knowledge of intact cord resuscitation, it seems illogical to cut the cord immediately and remove nonbreathing newborns from their only source of respiratory and circulatory support during this critical time [17,18].

We present a case of a moribund newborn who was successfully resuscitated with an intact cord and then discuss the probable physiology underlying this uncommon event. (see Figure 1) [2].

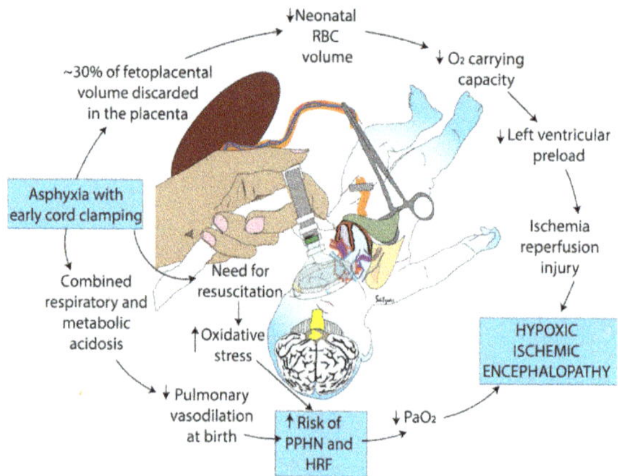

Figure 1. Negative consequences of early cord clamping in depressed infants who may have asphyxia and an increased need for resuscitation. Early cord clamping reduces whole blood and red blood cell (RBC) volume and increases the fetal blood left in the placenta. Hypovolemia and hypoxemia contribute to cerebral hypoperfusion and ischemia and exacerbate pulmonary hypoperfusion and hypertension. Studies have shown increased oxidative stress with early cord clamping compared to delayed cord clamping and umbilical cord milking. Oxidative stress contributes to ischemia and other neonatal morbidities such as hypoxic respiratory failure (HRF), hypoxic-ischemic encephalopathy and persistent pulmonary hypertension of the newborn (PPHN). Copyright Satyan Lakshminrusimha, MD, Sacramento, CA, USA. Used with permission [2].

2. Case Presentation

A 28-year-old woman having her second infant was in labor at term and progressed rapidly to full dilatation with intact membranes. During second stage, the baby's head remained high between contractions and recoiled after descending to the +3 station with each push. After artificial rupture of the membranes, the infant descended, crowned, and delivered in one contraction. A tight double nuchal cord was unwound immediately, and the cord was kept intact. The newborn was extremely pale white with no tone, reflexes, or respiratory effort and was placed on the bed between the mother's legs, where the provider bulb suctioned, dried, and stimulated the infant. A check of the heart rate at about 20 s revealed that it was over 100, the cord appeared full and pulsatile, and the infant was visibly gaining color. The provider continued to stimulate the baby with no response. At about 2 minutes (exact time was not recorded), the baby, now appearing well perfused, moved his left arm upon his chest, opened his eyes, took an easy breath, and quickly flexed his other extremities. The baby never vocalized a cry, even with strong stimulation, but continued gentle, even, and shallow respirations with clear lungs. The cord was clamped and cut about 20 minutes after birth, and the infant had a normal newborn course. At one year, the mother reported no concerns with the infant. (Adapted from case first published in Downe in 2008 [17]).

3. Discussion

Adequate circulation, as well as breathing, is essential for a successful neonatal transition. We are proposing the following points, which are illustrated in Figure 2. First, we discuss lung readiness in preparation for the initial breath and the importance of circulation as well as breathing for transition, and we describe how a placental transfusion may return blood volume to provide enhanced perfusion for all organs. Next, we provide evidence supporting our hypothesis that enhanced perfusion may stimulate the vagus nerve to cause vasodilation in the lung, thereby reducing pulmonary vascular resistance and increasing blood flow before the first breath. Last, we suggest that enhanced perfusion to the presented case infant's brain enabled breathing and establishment of consciousness, tone, and reflexes. Remaining attached to the umbilical cord after birth provided the infant full access to his fetal–placental blood volume to accomplish transition. Each point is described, explained, and referenced in the following text.

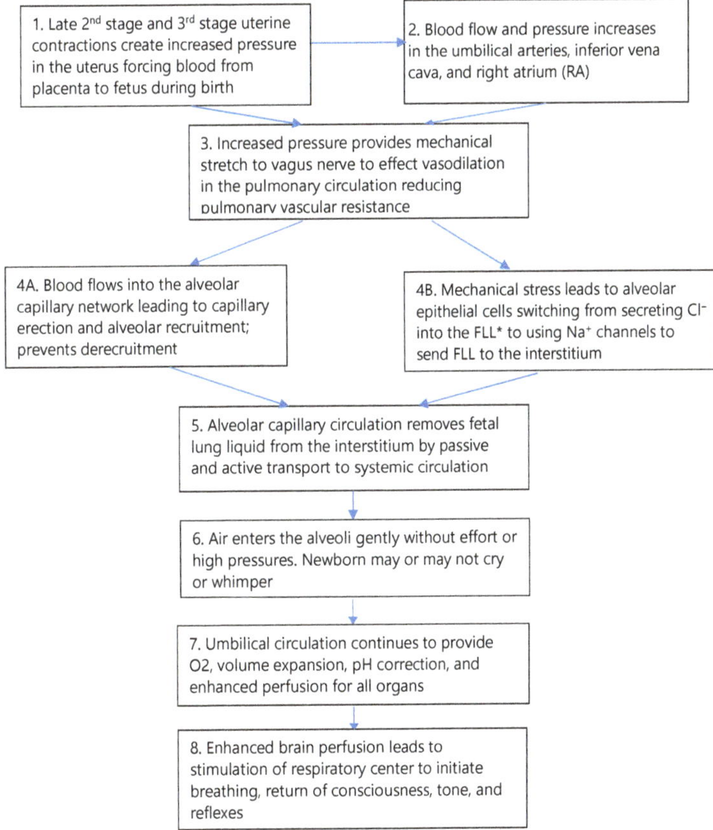

Figure 2. The blood volume model for physiologic neonatal transition.

3.1. Lung Readiness and Preparation for the First Breath

3.1.1. Lung Growth and Development in the Fetus

Lung growth in fetal life depends on the alveoli being highly distended with a large volume (20–30 mL/kg) of fetal lung liquid [20,21], which creates lung expansion along with mechanical stress/stretch that stimulates and promotes normal growth and development. If not for this liquid, the fetus would develop hypoplastic lungs [20]. The lungs maintain a low pH (6.27) in the alveolar fetal lung liquid constantly throughout fetal life [22]. It is important to clarify that fetal lung liquid is not amniotic fluid (Table 1) [20].

Table 1. Composition of Bodily Fluids Compared to Lung Fluid. * (mEq/L). Adapted from Plosa and Guttentag, Lung Development in Avery 10th Edition [20] and Bland R [22].

Component	Lung Fluid	Interstitial Fluid	Plasma	Amniotic Fluid
pH	6.27	7.31	7.34	7.02
Bicarbonate *	3	25	24	19
Protein (g/dL)	0.03	3.27	4.09	0.10
Sodium *	150	147	150	113
Potassium *	6.3	4.8	4.8	7.6
Chloride *	157	107	107	87

Fetal lung liquid is generated and maintained by the alveolar epithelial cells. These cells secrete chloride ions into the alveolar breathing spaces filled in utero with fetal lung liquid [22]. In most vascular beds, acidosis causes vasodilation. However, in the pulmonary circulation, acidosis evokes vasoconstriction supporting vascular resistance [23]. At birth, a switch must occur so that the alveolar epithelial cells stop secreting chloride into the fetal lung liquid and immediately begin to pump fetal lung liquid into the interstitium by means of sodium channels.

3.1.2. Anatomy of the Respiratory Tract and Blood Supply

The process of fetal lung liquid removal from the interstitium is informed by the anatomy of the alveolus and its blood supply [20]. About 80% of an adult's alveoli develop after birth. However, in the term newborn, around 50 million alveoli are covered by approximately 47 billion capillary segments [20] or a ratio of 1 alveolus to around 900 capillary segments. The capillaries are so dense that an almost continuous sheet of blood encircles each alveolus, allowing for maximal gas exchange. There is only a very thin (0.5 μm) interstitial space between an alveolus and the surrounding capillary network which facilitates gas exchange.

The large number of capillaries segments covering the alveoli are cemented to the alveoli by an extracellular matrix [24]. As the dense alveolar capillary network fills with blood, the capillary plexuses expand with blood and become erect [7,25,26]. This process opens the alveoli and provides the "scaffolding" structure that maintains alveolar expansion and likely prevents the alveoli from closing or collapsing on expiration [25,26].

The alveolar capillaries adapt to the sudden influx of blood at birth by increasing the diameter of the lumen, but they do not change the diameter of the capillary itself (Figure 3) [27,28]. This allows the overall lung volume to remain the same. Figure 3 shows the immediate decrease in wall thickness of the porcine pulmonary inter-acinar arteries as the lumens dilate with blood. This allows transfer and inflow of the blood that formerly circulated through the placenta for respiration during fetal life.

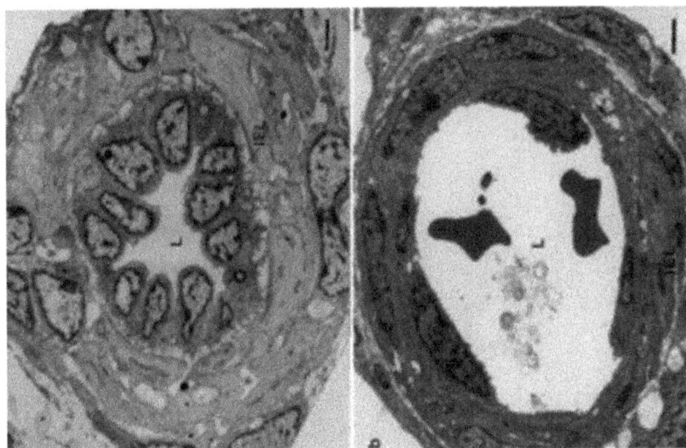

Figure 3. Electron micrographs of transverse sections through small muscular lung arterioles in naturally born piglets in a stillborn on the left and at 5 min of life taken at the same magnification. At birth, the endothelial cells of the intra-acinar arteries showed more rapid and greater changes in shape and thickness than did the cells of more proximal vessels. IEL: internal elastic lamina; L: lumen. Scale bar line on lower right = 2 μm. Adapted from Haworth et al. [27] (with permission).

3.1.3. Switching from Fetal to Neonatal Respiratory Function

At birth, the alveolar membrane makes an instantaneous switch from producing and maintaining the fetal lung liquid to excreting it to the interstitium [28]. We suggest that the mechanical stress/stretch from the reallotment of the residual placental blood volume into the alveolar capillary network plays a major role in the switch [22]. Perks et al., studying fetal goats at different gestational ages, found that lung expansion from the infusion of saline reduced production and reabsorption of fetal lung liquid [29]. They suggested that expansion of the lung activates the ion pump, Na^+/K^+-ATPase, which generates a transepithelial osmotic gradient that causes the movement of fluid out of the alveolar airspace to the interstitium [29]. It is likely that the enhanced vascular perfusion provides mechanical stress/stretch through vasodilation in the alveolar capillary network. This continues the distension, vital in fetal life, to support progressive neonatal lung development and growth [30]. Effects of the essential stretch over time on the vessels surrounding the alveoli can be seen in the porcine lung over the first five minutes (Figure 3) and hours (Figure 4) following normal birth [27,31].

After the switch, both Type I and II alveolar epithelial cells pump sodium ions out of the alveolar spaces into the interstitium, generating the driving force for removal of the fetal lung liquid from the alveoli rapidly after birth [22]. However, this fetal lung liquid cannot stay in the interstitium without compromising air exchange and requires rapid removal. The pulmonary circulation (alveolar capillary network) absorbs most of the residual fetal lung liquid from the interstitium after birth [22]. Thus, there are two rapid components to the process of fetal lung liquid removal: (1) transepithelial flow of the fetal lung liquid into the interstitium and (2) removal of the fetal lung liquid from the interstitium by the alveolar capillaries and into the systematic blood stream through the alveoli capillary network [22]. Evidence for the validity of the rapid removal of acidic fetal lung liquid is suggested by Wiberg's finding of a slight decrease in pH that has been reported in newborns with continued cord circulation [32,33]. The decrease in pH was significant in blood from the intact umbilical arteries at 45 s of life but not until after 90 s in the umbilical vein. This indicates that the newborn was the source of the change in pH and not the placenta. It was similar in infants born either vaginally or by cesarean section and occurred despite good oxygenation [32]. These findings show that the acidic fetal lung liquid must enter the infant's alveoli–capillary network blood supply rapidly. The change in pH is statistically, but not clinically, significant. However, for an infant with immediate or early cord clamping, the placental blood flow will not be available to assist with removal or dilution of the acidic lung liquid.

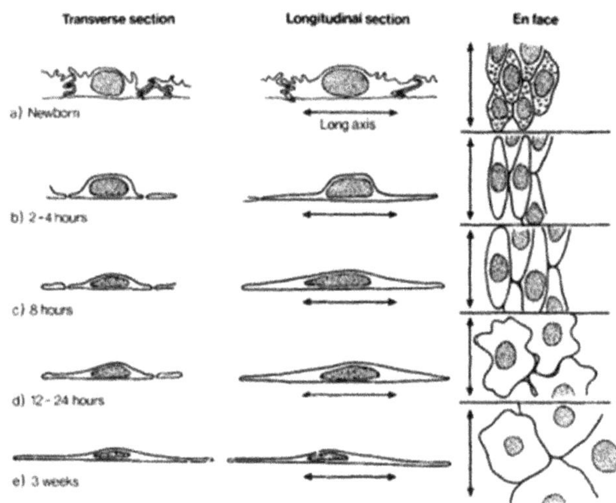

Figure 4. This diagram illustrates shape changes in the endothelial cells of intra-acinar arteries during the first 3 weeks of life (porcine). The endothelial cells of the intra-acinar arteries showed marked changes in cell shape and relationships after birth, while those of large preacinar arteries did not. The first structural changes detected during the first 30 min of life occurred in the endothelial cells lining the intra-acinar arteries. Adapted from Hall and Haworth [31] (with permission).

3.1.4. Breathing after Birth

The first breath our case newborn experienced does not fit the prevailing paradigm, which states that high initial negative pressure is required for lung opening to decrease the pulmonary vascular resistance at birth and push the lung fluid out of the alveolar spaces [34]. It is assumed that hypoxia will develop in the non-breathing infant, but in our case newborn, placental respiration overcame this as reflected in the newborn's heart rate and improving color. This is similar to the reliance of placental respiration and umbilical circulation during procedures using the ex-utero intrapartum technique (EXIT) [35]. The EXIT procedure consists of hysterotomy and partial delivery of the head and upper torso of the fetus while maintaining uteroplacental gas exchange from the umbilical cord. Normally, the procedure is said to be possible for 60 minutes, but cases with sufficient placental respiration and umbilical circulation for up to 150 minutes have been reported [36].

Recent studies report that applying a face mask or even nasal prongs to a newborn immediately after birth may inhibit initial breathing and reduce the heart rate [37–39]. Applying these devices induces vagally mediated facial reflexes that inhibit spontaneous breathing. The trigeminocardiac reflex and the laryngeal chemoreflex can also be elicited by air flow, leading to glottal closure [40]. Most likely, the mammalian diving reflex is triggered; it consists of breathing cessation (apnea), a dramatic slowing of the heart rate (bradycardia), and an increase in peripheral vasoconstriction. The diving reflex is thought to conserve vital oxygen stores and thus maintain life by directing perfusion to the two organs most essential for life: the heart and the brain [41].

A puzzling finding, given the current paradigm, is the report of reduced blood flow to the heart with breathing movements. A recent newborn lamb experiment found that the umbilical venous flow was markedly reduced with each breath [42]. In another newborn lamb study, a 30-s sustained inflation, even with delayed cord clamping, prevented the lamb's blood from flowing into the lung via the pulmonary artery and inferior vena cava [43]. A randomized control trial comparing sustained inflation with usual ventilation in human preterm infants was stopped because more early deaths occurred in the infants with sustained inflation [44].

These findings demonstrate that early or forced breaths may interfere with a physiologic transition by blocking the essential increased blood flow to the heart. Aerating the lung is critical for the success of neonatal transition but doing so before the lung has been adequately perfusion may be harmful. A heart rate above 100 or increasing indicates wellbeing and, as in our case, continued placental respiration [17]. Thus, attempting to start ventilation immediately after birth may compromise initial and early breathing as well as transition [45]. It is much easier to push air into lungs when the alveolar capillary circulation is fluid-filled [25,46].

Awareness of the heart rate allows a clinician to assess whether one can wait longer than one minute before assisting with ventilation. Waiting longer may be especially beneficial when there has been some cord compression as with a nuchal cord, shoulder dystocia, or occult cord. While some say that the main cause of persistent neonatal bradycardia is inadequate ventilation, we suggest that the loss of the available blood volume from immediate or early cord clamping is a likely cause in many cases. Bhatt has clearly demonstrated the cost of immediate cord clamping to the newborn by showing a 50% reduction in right ventricular output, heart rate, and pulmonary blood flow immediately after birth in preterm lambs [8]. Both Katheria and Nevill have reported that for preterm infants, there is no harm in waiting 60 s after birth to deliver the first assisted breath [2,47,48]. They found that 90% of the infants had breathed on their own by 60 s and that no clinical benefit was reported from assisted breathing before that time.

3.2. Circulation

3.2.1. Contents of Cord Blood

Maintenance of an intact cord allowed our case newborn to receive his full allotment of blood volume. This warm, oxygenated residual placenta blood amounts to about 15–20 mL/kg of red blood cells - enough to provide the term infant additional oxygen-carrying capacity and adequate iron for four to 12 months [49,50]. The blood also contains up to a billion of several kinds of stem cells providing an autologous transplant, which may reduce the neonate's susceptibility to both neonatal and age-related diseases [51]. Neuroprotective progesterone in the term neonate's blood at birth is almost two-times higher than the mother's level. It likely causes vasodilation, which can help to distribute the large amount of placental transfusion throughout the body [7,52,53]. In addition, this blood, unique in its composition for the newborn, contains many essential factors such as cytokines, growth factors, and important messengers that support and drive the process of transition (see Table 2) [11,54]. The enhanced perfusion provides higher pulmonary artery pressure [55] and mechanical stimuli, which causes electrochemical signaling that is likely essential for the normal function, maturation, and maintenance of all organs [7,30].

3.2.2. Placental Transfusion Enables the Return of Blood Volume

As the head is born and uterine fibers shorten, the uterus contracts with more pressure around the placenta. The strong expulsive contractions at the end of second stage or early third stage begin to force placental blood to the infant [56]. In humans, the intervals between these contractions allows for continued placental gas and nutrient exchange for the fetus/newborn [57,58]. Umbilical circulation continues to flow through the intact umbilical arteries for several minutes [59]. Boere measured the blood flow with doppler ultrasound in the intact umbilical cord of healthy term babies. Before cord clamping, over 80% of the infants in the study had umbilical arterial flow for a mean of four minutes, while almost half (43%) still had arterial flow when the cord was clamped at six minutes [59]. This information is not considered in current resuscitation protocols for infants of all gestational ages that imply immediate or early cord clamping and the care of the newborn away from the mother's bedside [2]. For our case infant, maintaining an intact cord was life-sustaining and likely avoided morbidity and possible mortality (Figure 1).

Table 2. Some components in cord blood and their role in the body. WBCs, white blood cells; ECs, endothelial cells. (Adapted from Chaudhury 2019; * Disdier 2018).

Factors/Messengers	Role
Angiopoietin	Vascular growth factor
Granulocyte-colony stimulating factor (G-CSF)	Stimulates bone marrow to make granulocytes and stem cells to release them
Bone morphogenic protein-9 (BMP-9)	Regulates iron metabolism; role in memory, learning, attention; bone formation
Endoglin (ENG)	Transmembrane glycoprotein in endothelial cells; growth factor; role in angiogenesis
Endothelian-1 (ET-1)	Peptide with key role in vascular homeostasis; vasoconstriction
Epidermal Growth Factor (EGF)	Transmembrane protein binding; cellular proliferation, differentiation, and survival
Interleukin-8 (IL-8)	Increases angiogenesis and phagocytosis; causes WBCs to migrate to site of injury; chemotaxis
Hepatic Growth Factor (HGF)	Morphogenic factor; paracrine cell growth motility
Heparin Binding EGF-like GF (HBEGF	Glycoprotein; role in heart development and function; would healing
Placental Growth Factor (PGF)	Role in angiogenesis and vasculogenesis
VEGF-A	Acts on ECs, increases vascular permeability, angio- and vasculogenesis, EC cell growth, cell migration; decreases apoptosis
Intra-Alpha inhibitor protein (IAIP) *	Provides anti-inflammatory neuroprotection; reduces production of reactive oxygen species *

3.2.3. Effect of Occlusion of the Umbilical Cord

Nuchal cord compression likely caused much of our case infant's blood volume to be sequestered in the placenta, resulting in the appearance of extreme paleness and unconsciousness [60]. Unwrapping the cord and leaving the cord intact allowed the blood that was sequestered in the placenta to reperfuse the infant's body so that he did not lose the essential blood volume necessary to oxygenate his brain and other vital organs. Although the cord felt pulseless initially, it began to pulse within 15 to 20 s, and the infant's body began to regain color.

When an umbilical vein is occluded, there is a possibility of a net transfer of blood from the fetus to the placenta (see Figure 5) [60]. The soft-walled vein can be compressed easily, preventing the return of blood volume to the fetus, while the more muscular-walled higher pressure arteries allow for a maintained flow from the fetus to the placenta. If severe enough, the loss of blood volume in the body can cause the fetus/newborn to appear to be unconsciousness and will result in extreme paleness at birth due to hypovolemia. Severe hypovolemia may lead to a sudden unexpected neonatal asystole, especially if the cord is severed immediately [60–62]. The neonatal status may be compromised by the uncorrected physiologic effects of blood volume loss leading to hypoxia.

3.3. Full Perfusion, the Vagus Nerve, and Pulmonary Vascular Resistance

One of the key features of the normal fetal-to-neonatal transition at birth is a reduction in the pulmonary vascular resistance to allow an increase in pulmonary blood flow. Credit has been given to lung aeration for decreasing the pulmonary vascular resistance at birth, although the mechanisms causing this have been debated for decades [63]. Surprisingly, Lang et al. found that severing the vagal nerve prevented the previously observed increase in pulmonary blood flow with partial lung aeration [64]. Compared to control newborn rabbits, he found that vagotomized rabbit newborns had little or no increase in pulmonary blood flow when ventilated with air or nitrogen gas. Using 100% oxygen for ventilation only partially mitigated the effect of the vagotomy. This new information suggests that the initial dramatic fall in pulmonary vascular resistance likely does not occur with ventilation/breathing alone but that vagal stimulation must play a significant role. Lang et al. suggests that given the importance of lowering the pulmonary vascular resistance, which is so essential to initiate blood flow to the lung, there are likely multiple overlapping mechanisms to ensure that this transition happens [64].

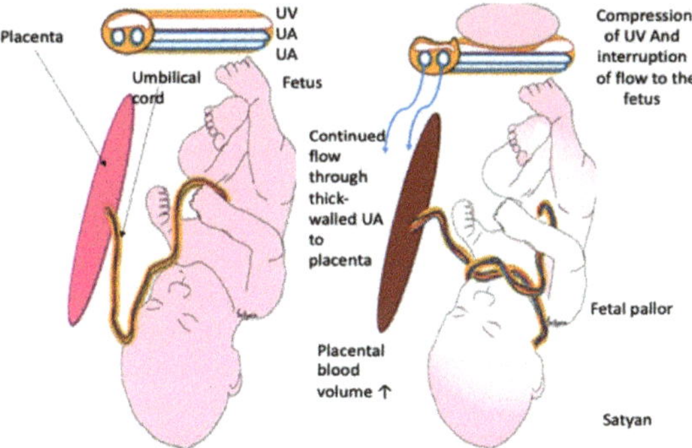

Figure 5. Effects of umbilical cord occlusion on the umbilical vein (UV) and umbilical arteries UA), placenta, and neonate. The "left figure" shows no occlusion; the "right figure" shows compression of the umbilical vein and interference with the flow from placenta to infant. Copyright by Satyan Lakshimrusimha, MD. Sacramento, CA, USA. Used with permission.

3.3.1. The Vagal Stimulation Hypothesis

The newborn illustrated in our case did not have any assisted breathing, and his first breaths were easy and quiet. The most plausible hypothesis for this is that enhanced perfusion from the placental transfusion stimulates the volume-sensing cardiopulmonary mechanisms [65]. As more blood volume enters the umbilical vein and moves through the inferior vena cava and into the right atrium, it signals the sinoatrial (SA) node (and other receptors) that blood flow is enhanced. The vagus nerve is stimulated via stretch mechanisms (baroreflex) to effect vasodilation in the lung, opening the pulmonary arteries and thus decreasing pulmonary vascular resistance [66]. This would have allowed blood flow into the alveolar capillary network supporting capillary erection, lung fluid removal, and likely an effortless first breath.

3.3.2. The Autonomic Nervous System

The autonomic nervous system is composed of two parts: the parasympathetic and sympathetic systems. Although their effects are opposed to each other, they work reciprocally to bring about the necessary responses to internal and external stimuli, continuously balancing each other to maintain homeostasis [67]. The vagal sensory input (part of the parasympathetic system) can detect visceral and environmental features and can adjust the central regulation of autonomic function to restore homeostasis. It can dampen the sympathetic activation to protect the oxygen-dependent central nervous system from the metabolically conservative defensive reactions (stress response, vasoconstriction, flight or fight, fainting).

In our featured case, decreased blood volume due to sequestration to the placenta likely reduced brain stem perfusion, thereby inhibiting consciousness, tone, and appropriate reflexes. When the compression of the cord was released immediately after birth and left intact, it allowed the placental residual blood to reallocate into the baby's body as validated by the robust pulsating cord. The returning blood volume distended the right heart's mechanical receptors, likely causing activation of the vagal complex to dilate the pulmonary arteries and the alveolar capillary network.

This idea is counter to the prevailing paradigm that it is the sympathetic nervous system that plays the predominant role in neonatal transition [68]. We suggest that soon after birth, the vagus nerve must dominate, as visceral homeostasis is incompatible with sympathetic domination [69]. It is important that the infant is not in a "fight or flight" response mode to initiate some of the first tasks after a successful transition (sucking and bonding). In the face of severe compromise, the fetus maintains autonomic nervous system function, which can be balanced with good perfusion [58].

3.4. Effects of Enhanced Perfusion on Consciousness, Breathing, Tone, and Reflexes

Impaired perfusion of the brainstem results in syncope, unconsciousness, decreased muscle tone, and lack of reflexes [70]. For our case newborn, the return of good perfusion to the heart and brain, sensed by various receptors in the body, resulted in domination of the vagal reflex, which reversed the negative changes of impaired perfusion. The return of tone and reflexes with breathing supports the idea that good perfusion of the brain is essential in an infant who appears unconscious and toneless at birth.

Our case newborn's one-minute Apgar score was two for a heart rate over 100. By two minutes of life, he opened his eyes and started easily breathing without assistance at the same time. The tone returned over his entire body, and he had good color and reflexes, resulting in a five-minute Apgar of 10. The case infant started breathing on his own without ventilation, gasping, or crying after his body was perfused. It is likely that some newborns receive at least some of their placental transfusion before they breathe for the first time, and this was clearly illustrated in our case [17,18]. The fetal–placental blood volume to the infant, from sustained cord circulation, supplies a higher level of systemic oxygen that stimulates the respiratory centers of the brain [68].

3.5. One Caveat: A Note of Caution

For an infant with an acute sequestration of blood in the placenta from cord compression, nuchal cord, or shoulder dystocia, the benefit from the return of this blood volume to the infant, via placental transfusion, is very important. However, there are a few infants for whom allowing for continued cord circulation may not make a difference. For those newborns, who may have had subtle chronic distress going on for hours during labor, the blood volume loss (mainly plasma) to the placenta may be significant. This can occur because of the fetal stress response during a difficult labor [58]. When a fetus is stressed, the blood pressure becomes elevated, and more of the fetus's blood reallocates to the placenta [71]. A transplacental water flux causes an increase in water loss from the fetus to the mother, reducing the fetus's total blood volume over time. Hypertonicity of contractions may be an important issue here as the fetus needs at least 1 or more minutes in between contractions to recover from the effects of the contractions and to prevent hypoxemia [58]. In a near-term sheep model, Brace reported a 7% blood volume loss from the fetus to the placenta in only 30 min by reducing the oxygen content for the near-term pregnant sheep. After returning the pregnant sheep to room air, it took about 30 min for the fetal blood volume to return to normal. However, in a few rare situations, there may not be enough blood volume left to assist in resuscitating the newborn. This mechanism as described by Brace needs further research [71].

4. Limitations

This article builds on many individual pieces of information obtained through careful human and animal research, which we incorporate to examine how bodily systems work together to accomplish the major life event of neonatal transition. While some of our conclusions are speculative, most are founded on solid physiologic principles and research. We cannot state the ideal time to clamp the cord, as it is not known. There is wide variety as to how long the arterial blood flow continues. We do not yet know if attachment to the low-resistance placenta may have a role in the prevention of neurologic or vascular issues. Optimal practice is likely to wait until the cord is flat and pale or until the placenta is ready to deliver.

5. Conclusions

We have presented a case of how intact cord resuscitation with sustained cord circulation supports transition. We have challenged many commonly held beliefs about neonatal resuscitation. The evidence suggests that the current practice of clamping and cutting the umbilical cord and moving the infant away from its mother and placenta is likely an unwise practice. Our case newborn, born depressed and non-vigorous, was fully resuscitated through maintenance of an intact cord. We believe that supporting the process of physiologic neonatal transition may avert potential morbidity or mortality. Placing an emphasis on full perfusion for the neonate after birth may help ensure further advancements in the prevention and treatment of conditions such as ischemic hypoxic encephalopathy and neurodevelopmental injury for infants of all gestational ages.

Author Contributions: Conceptualization, J.M.; writing—original draft preparation, J.M.; writing—review and editing, J.M., D.E.-O., K.J., H.R. and O.A. All authors have read and agreed to the published version of the manuscript.

Funding: This research received no external funding.

Acknowledgments: We are very grateful to Susan Bewley for review and critique of the manuscript and her suggestions for improvement.

Conflicts of Interest: The authors declare no conflict of interest.

References

1. Aziz, K.; Lee, H.C.; Escobedo, M.B.; Hoover, A.V.; Kamath-Rayne, B.D.; Kapadia, V.S.; Magid, D.J.; Niermeyer, S.; Schmölzer, G.M.; Szyld, E.; et al. Part 5: Neonatal Resuscitation 2020 American Heart Association Guidelines for Cardiopulmonary Resuscitation and Emergency Cardiovascular Care. *Pediatrics* **2021**, *147*, e2020038505E. [CrossRef] [PubMed]
2. Katheria, A.C.; Rich, W.D.; Bava, S.; Lakshminrusimha, S. Placental Transfusion for Asphyxiated Infants. *Front. Pediatr.* **2019**, *7*, 473. [CrossRef] [PubMed]
3. Backes, C.H.; Rivera, B.K.; Haque, U.; Bridge, J.A.; Smith, C.V.; Hutchon, D.J.R.; Mercer, J.S. Placental Transfusion Strategies in Very Preterm Neonates. *Obstet. Gynecol.* **2014**, *124*, 47–56. [CrossRef]
4. Fogarty, M.; Osborn, D.A.; Askie, L.; Seidler, A.L.; Hunter, K.; Lui, K.; Simes, J.; Tarnow-Mordi, W. Delayed vs early umbilical cord clamping for preterm infants: A systematic review and meta-analysis. *Am. J. Obstet. Gynecol.* **2018**, *218*, 1–18. [CrossRef] [PubMed]
5. Rabe, H.; Gyte, G.M.; Díaz-Rossello, J.L.; Duley, L. Effect of timing of umbilical cord clamping and other strategies to influence placental transfusion at preterm birth on maternal and infant outcomes. *Cochrane Database Syst. Rev.* **2019**, *9*, CD003248. [CrossRef]
6. Robledo, K.P.; O Tarnow-Mordi, W.; Rieger, I.; Suresh, P.; Martin, A.; Yeung, C.; Ghadge, A.; Liley, H.G.; Osborn, D.; Morris, J.; et al. Effects of delayed versus immediate umbilical cord clamping in reducing death or major disability at 2 years corrected age among very preterm infants (APTS): A multicentre, randomised clinical trial. *Lancet Child Adolesc. Health* **2022**, *6*, 150–157. [CrossRef]
7. Mercer, J.S.; Erickson-Owens, D.A.; Rabe, H. Placental transfusion: May the "force" be with the baby. *J. Perinatol.* **2021**, *41*, 1495–1504. [CrossRef]
8. Bhatt, S.; Polglase, G.; Wallace, E.; Pas, A.T.; Hooper, S.B. Ventilation before Umbilical Cord Clamping Improves the Physiological Transition at Birth. *Front. Pediatr.* **2014**, *2*, 113. [CrossRef]
9. Kc, A.; Singhal, N.; Gautam, J.; Rana, N.; Andersson, O. Effect of early versus delayed cord clamping in neonate on heart rate, breathing and oxygen saturation during first 10 minutes of birth—Randomized clinical trial. *Matern. Health Neonatol. Perinatol.* **2019**, *5*, 7. [CrossRef]
10. Yao, A. Lind, Distribution of blood between infant and placenta after birth. *Lancet* **1969**, *2*, 871–873. [CrossRef]
11. Chaudhury, S.; Saqibuddin, J.; Birkett, R.; Falcon-Girard, K.; Kraus, M.; Ernst, L.M.; Grobman, W.; Mestan, K.K. Variations in Umbilical Cord Hematopoietic and Mesenchymal Stem Cells with Bronchopulmonary Dysplasia. *Front. Pediatr.* **2019**, *7*, 475. [CrossRef] [PubMed]
12. Badurdeen, S.; Roberts, C.; Blank, D.; Miller, S.; Stojanovska, V.; Davis, P.; Hooper, S.; Polglase, G. Haemodynamic Instability and Brain Injury in Neonates Exposed to Hypoxia–Ischaemia. *Brain Sci.* **2019**, *9*, 49. [CrossRef] [PubMed]
13. Katheria, A.; Hosono, S.; El-Naggar, W. A new wrinkle: Umbilical cord management (how, when, who). *Semin. Fetal Neonatal Med.* **2018**, *23*, 321–326. [CrossRef] [PubMed]
14. Andersson, O.; Rana, N.; Ewald, U.; Målqvist, M.; Stripple, G.; Basnet, O.; Subedi, K.; Kc, A. Intact cord resuscitation versus early cord clamping in the treatment of depressed newborn infants during the first 10 minutes of birth (Nepcord III)—A randomized clinical trial. *Matern. Health Neonatol. Perinatol.* **2019**, *5*, 15. [CrossRef]
15. Isacson, M.; Gurung, R.; Basnet, O.; Andersson, O.; Kc, A. Neurodevelopmental outcomes of a randomised trial of intact cord resuscitation. *Acta Paediatr.* **2021**, *110*, 465–472. [CrossRef]
16. Polglase, G.R.; Schmölzer, G.M.; Roberts, C.; Blank, D.A.; Badurdeen, S.; Crossley, K.J.; Miller, S.L.; Stojanovska, V.; Galinsky, R.; Kluckow, M.; et al. Cardiopulmonary Resuscitation of Asystolic Newborn Lambs Prior to Umbilical Cord Clamping; the Timing of Cord Clamping Matters! *Front. Physiol.* **2020**, *11*, 902. [CrossRef]

17. Mercer, J.; Erickson-Owens, D.; Skovgaard, R. Fetal to Neonatal Transition: First, Do No Harm. In *Normal Birth*, 2nd ed.; Churchill Livingstone Elsevier: Edinburgh, Scotland, 2008; pp. 149–174.

18. Fulton, C.; Stoll, K.; Thordarson, D. Bedside resuscitation of newborns with an intact umbilical cord: Experiences of midwives from British Columbia. *Midwifery* **2016**, *34*, 42–46. [CrossRef]

19. Downey, C.L.; Bewley, S. Historical perspectives on umbilical cord clamping and neonatal transition. *J. R. Soc. Med.* **2012**, *105*, 325–329. [CrossRef]

20. Plosa, E.; Guttentag, S.H. Lung Development. In *Avery's Diseases of the Newborn*, 10th ed.; Elsevie: Philadephia, PA, USA, 2018; pp. 586–599.

21. Hooper, S.B.; Harding, R. Harding, Fetal lung liquid: A major determinant of the growth and functional development of the fetal lung. *Clin. Exp. Pharmacol. Physiol.* **1995**, *22*, 235–247. [CrossRef]

22. Bland, R.D. Lung Fluid Balance During Development. *NeoReviews* **2005**, *6*, e255–e267. [CrossRef]

23. Lumb, A.; Slinger, P. Hypoxic Pulmonary Vasoconstriction. *Anesthesiology* **2015**, *122*, 932–946. [CrossRef] [PubMed]

24. Zhou, Y.; Horowitz, J.C.; Naba, A.; Ambalavanan, N.; Atabai, K.; Balestrini, J.; Bitterman, P.B.; Corley, R.A.; Ding, B.-S.; Engler, A.J.; et al. Extracellular matrix in lung development, homeostasis and disease. *Matrix Biol.* **2018**, *73*, 77–104. [CrossRef] [PubMed]

25. Jaykka, S. Capillary erection and the structural appearance of fetal and neonatl lungs. *Acta Paediatr.* **1958**, *47*, 484–500. [CrossRef] [PubMed]

26. Mercer, J.S.; Skovgaard, R.L. Neonatal Transitional Physiology. *J. Périnat. Neonatal Nurs.* **2002**, *15*, 56–75. [CrossRef] [PubMed]

27. Haworth, S.G.; Hall, S.M.; Chew, M.; Allen, K. Thinning of fetal pulmonary arterial wall and postnatal remodeling: Ultrastructural studies on the respiratory unit arteries of the pig. *Virchows Arch A* **1987**, *411*, 161–171. [CrossRef] [PubMed]

28. Gao, Y.; Raj, J.U. Regulation of the Pulmonary Circulation in the Fetus and Newborn. *Physiol. Rev.* **2010**, *90*, 1291–1335. [CrossRef]

29. Perks, A.M.; Cassin, S. The rate of production of lung liquid in fetal goats, and the effect of expansion of the lungs. *J. Dev. Physiol.* **1985**, *7*, 149–160.

30. Lorenz, L.; Axnick, J.; Buschmann, T.; Henning, C.; Urner, S.; Fang, S.; Nurmi, H.; Eichhorst, N.; Holtmeier, R.; Bódis, K.; et al. Mechanosensing by β1 integrin induces angiocrine signals for liver growth and survival. *Nature* **2018**, *562*, 128–132. [CrossRef]

31. Hall, S.M.; Haworth, S.G. Normal adaptation of pulmonary arterial intima to extrauterine life in the pig: Ultrastructural studies. *J. Pathol.* **1986**, *149*, 55–66. [CrossRef]

32. Giovannini, N.; Crippa, B.L.; Denaro, E.; Raffaeli, G.; Cortesi, V.; Consonni, D.; Cetera, G.E.; Parazzini, F.; Ferrazzi, E.; Mosca, F.; et al. The effect of delayed umbilical cord clamping on cord blood gas analysis in vaginal and caesarean-delivered term newborns without fetal distress: A prospective observational study. *BJOG Int. J. Obstet. Gynaecol.* **2020**, *127*, 405–413. [CrossRef]

33. Wiberg, N.; Källén, K.; Olofsson, P. Delayed umbilical cord clamping at birth has effects on arterial and venous blood gases and lactate concentrations. *BJOG Int. J. Obstet. Gynaecol.* **2008**, *115*, 697–703. [CrossRef] [PubMed]

34. Lara-Cantón, I.; Badurdeen, S.; Dekker, J.; Davis, P.; Roberts, C.; Pas, A.T.; Vento, M. Oxygen saturation and heart rate in healthy term and late preterm infants with delayed cord clamping. *Pediatr. Res.* 2022; epub ahead of print. [CrossRef]

35. Spiers, A.; Legendre, G.; Biquard, F.; Descamps, P.; Corroenne, R. Ex Utero Intrapartum Technique (EXIT): Indications, procedure methods and materno-fetal complications – A literature review. *J. Gynecol. Obstet. Hum. Reprod.* **2022**, *51*, 102252. [CrossRef]

36. Hirose, S.; Sydorak, R.M.; Tsao, K.; Cauldwell, C.B.; Newman, K.D.; Mychaliska, G.; Albanese, C.T.; Lee, H.; Farmer, D. Spectrum of intrapartum management strategies for giant fetal cervical teratoma. *J. Pediatr. Surg.* **2003**, *38*, 446–450. [CrossRef] [PubMed]

37. Kuypers, K.L.; Lamberska, T.; Martherus, T.; Dekker, J.; Böhringer, S.; Hooper, S.B.; Plavka, R.; Pas, A.B.T. The effect of a face mask for respiratory support on breathing in preterm infants at birth. *Resuscitation* **2019**, *144*, 178–184. [CrossRef] [PubMed]

38. Kuypers, K.; Martherus, T.; Lamberska, T.; Dekker, J.; Hooper, S.B.; Pas, A.B.T. Reflexes that impact spontaneous breathing of preterm infants at birth: A narrative review. *Arch. Dis. Child. Fetal Neonatal Ed.* **2020**, *105*, 675–679. [CrossRef]

39. Gaertner, V.D.; Rüegger, C.M.; O'Currain, E.; Kamlin, C.O.F.; Hooper, S.B.; Davis, P.G.; Springer, L. Physiological responses to facemask application in newborns immediately after birth. *Arch. Dis. Child. Fetal Neonatal Ed.* **2021**, *106*, 381–385. [CrossRef]

40. Dekker, J.; van Kaam, A.H.; Roehr, C.C.; Flemmer, A.W.; Foglia, E.E.; Hooper, S.B.; Pas, A.B.T. Stimulating and maintaining spontaneous breathing during transition of preterm infants. *Pediatr. Res.* **2021**, *90*, 722–730. [CrossRef]

41. Panneton, W.M.; Gan, Q. The Mammalian Diving Response: Inroads to Its Neural Control. *Front. Neurosci.* **2020**, *14*, 524. [CrossRef]

42. Brouwer, E.; Pas, A.B.T.; Polglase, G.R.; McGillick, E.; Böhringer, S.; Crossley, K.J.; Rodgers, K.; Blank, D.; Yamaoka, S.; Gill, A.W.; et al. Effect of spontaneous breathing on umbilical venous blood flow and placental transfusion during delayed cord clamping in preterm lambs. *Arch. Dis. Child. Fetal Neonatal Ed.* **2020**, *105*, 26–32. [CrossRef]

43. Nair, J.; Davidson, L.; Gugino, S.; Koenigsknecht, C.; Helman, J.; Nielsen, L.; Sankaran, D.; Agrawal, V.; Chandrasekharan, P.; Rawat, M.; et al. Sustained Inflation Reduces Pulmonary Blood Flow during Resuscitation with an Intact Cord. *Children* **2021**, *8*, 353. [CrossRef]

44. Kirpalani, H.; Ratcliffe, S.; Keszler, M.; Davis, P.G.; Foglia, E.E.; Pas, A.T.; Fernando, M.; Chaudhary, A.; Localio, R.; Van Kaam, A.H.; et al. Effect of Sustained Inflations vs Intermittent Positive Pressure Ventilation on Bronchopulmonary Dysplasia or Death Among Extremely Preterm Infants. *JAMA* **2019**, *321*, 1165–1175. [CrossRef] [PubMed]

45. Claassen, C.C.; Strand, M.L. Understanding the Risks and Benefits of Delivery Room CPAP for Term Infants. *Pediatrics* **2019**, *144*, e20191720. [CrossRef] [PubMed]

46. Avery, M.E.; Frank, N.R.; Gribetz, I. The inflationary force produced by pulmonary vascular distension in excised lungs. *J. Clin. Investig.* **1959**, *38*, 456–462. [CrossRef]
47. Katheria, A.C.; Brown, M.K.; Faksh, A.; Hassen, K.O.; Rich, W.; Lazarus, D.; Steen, J.; Daneshmand, S.S.; Finer, N.N. Delayed Cord Clamping in Newborns Born at Term at Risk for Resuscitation: A Feasibility Randomized Clinical Trial. *J. Pediatr.* **2017**, *187*, 313–317.e1. [CrossRef] [PubMed]
48. Meyer, M.; Nevill, E. The Assisted Breathing before Cord Clamping (ABC) Study Protocol. *Children* **2021**, *8*, 336. [CrossRef]
49. Dewey, K.G.; Chaparro, C.M. Session 4: Mineral metabolism and body composition Iron status of breast-fed infants. *Proc. Nutr. Soc.* **2007**, *66*, 412–422. [CrossRef]
50. Andersson, O.; Mercer, J.S. Cord Management of the Term Newborn. *Clin. Perinatol.* **2021**, *48*, 447–470. [CrossRef]
51. Borlongan, C.V.; Lawton, C.; Acosta, S.; Watson, N.; Gonzales-Portillo, C.; Diamandis, T.; Tajiri, N.; Kaneko, Y.; Sanberg, P.R. Enhancing endogenous stem cells in the newborn via delayed umbilical cord clamping. *Neural Regen. Res.* **2015**, *10*, 1359–1362. [CrossRef]
52. González-Orozco, J.C.; Camacho-Arroyo, I. Progesterone Actions During Central Nervous System Development. *Front. Neurosci.* **2019**, *13*, 503. [CrossRef]
53. Sippell, W.G.; Becker, H.; Versmold, H.T.; Bidlingmaier, F.; Knorr, D. Longitudinal Studies of Plasma Aldosterone, Corticosterone, Deoxycorticosterone, Progesterone, 17-Hydroxyprogesterone, Cortisol, and Cortisone Determined Simultaneously in Mother and Child at Birth and during the Early Neonatal Period. I. Spontaneous Delivery. *J. Clin. Endocrinol. Metab.* **1978**, *46*, 971–985. [CrossRef]
54. Disdier, C.; Zhang, J.; Fukunaga, Y.; Lim, Y.; Qiu, J.; Santoso, A.; Stonestreet, B.S. Alterations in inter-alpha inhibitor protein expression after hypoxic-ischemic brain injury in neonatal rats. *Int. J. Dev. Neurosci.* **2018**, *65*, 54–60. [CrossRef] [PubMed]
55. Arcilla, R.A.; Oh, W.; Lind, J.; Gessner, I.H. Pulmonary Arterial Pressures of Newborn Infants Born with Early and Late Clamping of the Cord. *Acta Paediatr.* **1966**, *55*, 305–315. [CrossRef] [PubMed]
56. Caldeyro, R.; Alvarez, H.; Reynolds, S.R.M. Reynolds, A better understanding of uterine contractility through simultaneous recording with an internal and a seven channel external method. *Obstet. Gynecol. Surv.* **1950**, *91*, 641–650. [CrossRef]
57. Hutchon, D.; Pratesi, S.; Katheria, A. How to Provide Motherside Neonatal Resuscitation with Intact Placental Circulation? *Children* **2021**, *8*, 291. [CrossRef] [PubMed]
58. Lear, C.A.; Galinsky, R.; Wassink, G.; Yamaguchi, K.; Davidson, J.; Westgate, J.A.; Bennet, L.; Gunn, A.J. The myths and physiology surrounding intrapartum decelerations: The critical role of the peripheral chemoreflex. *J. Physiol.* **2016**, *594*, 4711–4725. [CrossRef]
59. Boere, I.; Roest, A.A.W.; Wallace, E.; Harkel, A.D.J.T.; Haak, M.C.; Morley, C.; Hooper, S.B.; Pas, A.T. Umbilical blood flow patterns directly after birth before delayed cord clamping. *Arch. Dis. Child. Fetal Neonatal Ed.* **2015**, *100*, F121–F125. [CrossRef]
60. Mercer, J.; Erickson-Owens, D.; Skovgaard, R. Cardiac asystole at birth: Is hypovolemic shock the cause? *Med. Hypotheses* **2009**, *72*, 458–463. [CrossRef]
61. Menticoglou, S.; Schneider, C. Resuscitating the Baby after Shoulder Dystocia. *Case Rep. Obstet. Gynecol.* **2016**, *2016*, 8674167. [CrossRef]
62. Ancora, G.; Meloni, C.; Soffritti, S.; Sandri, F.; Ferretti, E. Intrapartum Asphyxiated Newborns Without Fetal Heart Rate and Cord Blood Gases Abnormalities: Two Case Reports of Shoulder Dystocia to Reflect Upon. *Front. Pediatr.* **2020**, *8*, 570332. [CrossRef]
63. Polglase, G.; Kluckow, M.; Gill, A.; Hooper, S. Hemodynamics of the Circulatory Transition. In *Hypoxic Respiratory Failure in the Newborn: From Origins to Clinical Management*, 1st ed.; CRC Press: Boca Raton, FL, USA, 2021; pp. 57–60.
64. Lang, J.A.R.; Pearson, J.T.; Binder-Heschl, C.; Wallace, M.J.; Siew, M.L.; Kitchen, M.; Pas, A.T.; Lewis, R.A.; Polglase, G.R.; Shirai, M.; et al. Vagal denervation inhibits the increase in pulmonary blood flow during partial lung aeration at birth. *J. Physiol.* **2017**, *595*, 1593–1606. [CrossRef]
65. Segar, J.L. Ontogeny of the arterial and cardiopulmonary baroreflex during fetal and postnatal life. *Am. J. Physiol. Content* **1997**, *273*, R457–R471. [CrossRef] [PubMed]
66. Barbeau, S.; Gilbert, G.; Cardouat, G.; Baudrimont, I.; Freund-Michel, V.; Guibert, C.; Marthan, R.; Vacher, P.; Quignard, J.-F.; Ducret, T. Mechanosensitivity in Pulmonary Circulation: Pathophysiological Relevance of Stretch-Activated Channels in Pulmonary Hypertension. *Biomolecules* **2021**, *11*, 1389. [CrossRef] [PubMed]
67. Drew, R.C.; Sinoway, L.I. Autonomic Control of the Heart. In *Primer on Autonomic Nervous System*, 3rd ed.; Elsivier: New York, NY, USA, 2012; pp. 177–180.
68. Mulkey, S.B.; Plessis, A.D. The Critical Role of the Central Autonomic Nervous System in Fetal-Neonatal Transition. *Semin. Pediatr. Neurol.* **2018**, *28*, 29–37. [CrossRef] [PubMed]
69. Porges, S.W. Cardiac vagal tone: A neurophysiological mechanism that evolved in mammals to dampen threat reactions and promote sociality. *World Psychiatry* **2021**, *20*, 296–298. [CrossRef]
70. McIntyre, S.; Nelson, K.; Mulkey, S.; Lechpammer, M.; Molloy, E.; Badawi, N. Neonatal encephalopathy: Focus on epidemiology and underexplored aspects of etiology. *Semin. Fetal Neonatal Med.* **2021**, *26*, 101265. [CrossRef]
71. Brace, R.A. Fetal blood volume responses to acute fetal hypoxia. *Am. J. Obstet. Gynecol.* **1986**, *155*, 889–893. [CrossRef]

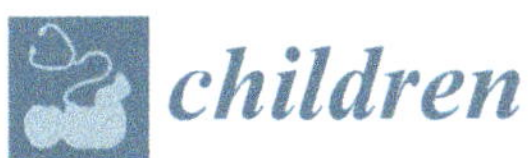

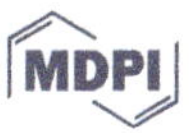

Article

Resuscitation with an Intact Cord Enhances Pulmonary Vasodilation and Ventilation with Reduction in Systemic Oxygen Exposure and Oxygen Load in an Asphyxiated Preterm Ovine Model

Praveen Chandrasekharan [1,*], Sylvia Gugino [1], Justin Helman [1], Carmon Koenigsknecht [1], Lori Nielsen [1], Nicole Bradley [1], Jayasree Nair [1], Vikash Agrawal [2], Mausma Bawa [1], Andreina Mari [1], Munmun Rawat [1] and Satyan Lakshminrusimha [3]

[1] Department of Pediatrics, Jacobs School of Medicine & Biomedical Sciences, University at Buffalo, Buffalo, NY 14260, USA; sfgugino@buffalo.edu (S.G.); jhelman@buffalo.edu (J.H.); carmonko@buffalo.edu (C.K.); lnielsen@buffalo.edu (L.N.); nkbradle@buffalo.edu (N.B.); jnair2@buffalo.edu (J.N.); mausmaba@buffalo.edu (M.B.); amaritor@buffalo.edu (A.M.); mrawat@upa.chob.edu (M.R.)

[2] Department of Pediatrics, Loma Linda University, Loma Linda, CA 92350, USA; dragrawalmd@gmail.com

[3] Department of Pediatrics, Division of Neonatology, University of California Davis School of Medicine, Sacramento, CA 95817, USA; slakshmi@ucdavis.edu

* Correspondence: pkchandr@buffalo.edu

Citation: Chandrasekharan, P.; Gugino, S.; Helman, J.; Koenigsknecht, C.; Nielsen, L.; Bradley, N.; Nair, J.; Agrawal, V.; Bawa, M.; Torrealba, A.M.; et al. Resuscitation with an Intact Cord Enhances Pulmonary Vasodilation and Ventilation with Reduction in Systemic Oxygen Exposure and Oxygen Load in an Asphyxiated Preterm Ovine Model. *Children* **2021**, *8*, 307. https://doi.org/10.3390/children8040307

Academic Editor: Simone Pratesi

Received: 1 April 2021
Accepted: 15 April 2021
Published: 17 April 2021

Abstract: (1) Background: Optimal initial oxygen (O_2) concentration in preterm neonates is controversial. Our objectives were to compare the effect of delayed cord clamping with ventilation (DCCV) to early cord clamping followed by ventilation (ECCV) on O_2 exposure, gas exchange, and hemodynamics in an asphyxiated preterm ovine model. (2) Methods: Asphyxiated preterm lambs (127–128 d) with heart rate <90 bpm were randomly assigned to DCCV or ECCV. In DCCV, positive pressure ventilation (PPV) was initiated with 30–60% O_2 and titrated based on preductal saturations (SpO_2) with an intact cord for 5 min, followed by clamping. In ECCV, the cord was clamped, and PPV was initiated. (3) Results: Fifteen asphyxiated preterm lambs were randomized to DCCV (N = 7) or ECCV (N = 8). The inspired O_2 (40 ± 20% vs. 60 ± 20%, $p < 0.05$) and oxygen load (520 (IQR 414–530) vs. 775 (IQR 623–868), p-0.03) in the DCCV group were significantly lower than ECCV. Arterial oxygenation and carbon dioxide ($PaCO_2$) levels were significantly lower and peak pulmonary blood flow was higher with DCCV. (4) Conclusion: In asphyxiated preterm lambs, resuscitation with an intact cord decreased O_2 exposure load improved ventilation with an increase in peak pulmonary blood flow in the first 5 min.

Keywords: delayed cord clamping; oxygen exposure; preterm neonates

1. Introduction

In the delivery room, a depressed preterm neonate often needs positive pressure ventilation (PPV) with supplemental oxygen [1]. In a surfactant deficient state complicated by birth asphyxia, the current recommendations to start ventilation with 21–30% oxygen (O_2) may not achieve target saturations (SpO_2) [2–4]. Inability to achieve target SpO_2 by 5 min is associated with poor outcomes in preterm infants. Birth asphyxia could increase pulmonary vascular resistance (PVR) and impair pulmonary vascular transition at birth. In a subgroup analysis of the Targeted Oxygen in the Resuscitation of Preterm Infants and their Developmental Outcomes (To2rpido) trial by Oei et al. <28-week gestation preterm infants resuscitated with 21% O_2 had higher mortality due to respiratory failure, compared to 100% O_2 [5]. Previously, we have shown that ventilation with 100% O_2 (but not 21%), led to a decrease in PVR and increased systemic to pulmonary pressure gradient in preterm lambs [6]. Such impaired pulmonary vascular transition at birth could explain the higher mortality demonstrated by Oei et al. in <28-week infants resuscitated with 21% oxygen [5]. Although 100% O_2 exposure in preterm lambs was associated with improved pulmonary blood flow and preductal SpO_2, it also led to supraphysiological arterial oxygenation (PaO_2) that could lead to hyperoxic injury [6]. With concerns of hyperoxia, higher oxidative injury, the use of 100% O_2 is not recommended [2,3].

The feasibility of delaying the clamping of the cord and its benefits have been studied extensively [1,7–15]. However, optimal oxygenation during delayed cord claming (DCC) and ventilation is not known. Ventilation with an intact cord has been shown to improve cardiovascular transition in both translational animal models and human newborns [10–13,15–24]. It has been recently reported that the preductal SpO_2 in neonates who had an intact cord was higher compared to the recommended SpO_2 ranges obtained following early cord clamping (ECC) [13,16,22].

Currently, there are no concrete recommendations to delay the clamping of the cord and provide positive pressure ventilation in a depressed preterm neonate [2,3]. We conducted this pilot study to understand the effect of ventilation and supplemental oxygen with an intact cord using an asphyxiated preterm ovine model to address this knowledge gap. We aimed to study the effect of supplementing oxygen with and without an intact cord in the setting of perinatal acidosis, on preductal SpO_2, oxygenation, ventilation, and hemodynamic parameters in the first 5 min of resuscitation.

2. Materials and Methods

The study was approved by the Institutional Animal Care and Use Committee, University of Buffalo, Buffalo New York, USA and followed the ARRIVE guidelines. Time-dated ewes (127–128 d, gestation), approximately equivalent in lung maturity to preterm neonate $\approx$28-week gestation were used in this study. The ewes did not receive antenatal steroids. After an overnight fast, the ewes were anesthetized, a caesarean section was performed, and fetal lambs were partially exteriorized. These fetal lambs were instrumented while in placental circulation as described previously [6]. Instrumentation included placement of the right jugular and carotid lines for access, pressure monitoring, and blood draws. A left carotid artery probe was placed to monitor blood flows. The left pulmonary artery probe and ductal arteriosus probe were placed to monitor blood flows. The lambs were intubated, and the lung fluid was drained by gravity.

Asphyxia was induced by umbilical cord occlusion until the heart rate (HR) reached <90 bpm. Once the target HR was achieved, the fetus was randomized to early cord clamping and ventilation (ECCV) or delayed cord clamping and ventilation (DCCV) for 5 min. Our primary objective was to achieve a composite outcome of HR $\geq$100 bpm and SpO_2 $\geq$80% by 5 min. For this reason, in DCCV, the cord was clamped only after 5 min unless the fetus had a drop in HR <60 bpm and ventilation continued. To simulate a real-life clinical scenario, the initial supplemental oxygen (O_2) concentration was between 30–60% in both groups and not changed during the first 2 min of PPV. After 2 min, the O_2 concentration was adjusted based on the neonatal resuscitation program (NRP) recommended target preductal SpO_2. The titration of O_2 was proportional to the difference between observed SpO_2 and target SpO_2 and was performed every min. In order to obtain an accurate and continuous recording of preductal SpO_2, two preductal probes (on the tongue and the right upper limb) were placed.

Oxygen load (OL) was calculated using the following formula, OL = (VT $\times$ FiO$_2$)/kg, where VT is tidal volume and FiO$_2$ is a fraction of inspired oxygen. Total OL was calculated using the summation of breaths for 5 min as defined previously [25].

In a depressed, asphyxiated and surfactant-deficient preterm lamb with HR < 90 bpm, our primary objective was to evaluate if titrating supplemental O_2 with (DCCV) and without an intact cord (ECCV) would lead to a higher rate of success in achieving target saturations as recommended by neonatal resuscitation program (NRP). The secondary objectives were to assess gas exchange and systemic and pulmonary hemodynamics along with oxygen load in the first 5 min of resuscitation.

Parametric data are presented as mean and standard deviation and analyzed by ANOVA. Non-parametric data are presented as median and interquartile range and analyzed by the Kruskal-Wallis test. The significance was set at a probability of less than five percent.

3. Results

Fifteen preterm lambs were randomized to DCCV (N-7) and ECCV (N-8). The characteristics are shown in Table 1 and were similar.

Table 1. Characteristics of preterm lambs.

Characteristics	ECC + V (N = 8)	DCC + V (N = 7)
Gestational age (days)	127 ± 0.52	128 ± 0.84
Female (N)	4	3
Birth weight (kg)	3.3 ± 0.63	3.3 ± 0.70
Born by multiplicity (N)	Twin–6	Twin–4
Heart rate at asphyxia (bpm)	88 ± 8	86 ± 10
Mean blood pressure at asphyxia (mmHg)	36 ± 8	34 ± 10
pH before resuscitation	7.04 ± 0.08	7.0 ± 0.08
$PaCO_2$ before resuscitation (mmHg)	90 ± 25	101 ± 23
PaO_2 before resuscitation (mmHg)	14 ± 6	15 ± 11

Data presented as numbers or as average and standard deviation. ECC—early cord clamping, DCC—delayed cord clamping, V—ventilation. $PaCO_2$—arterial carbon dioxide, PaO_2—arterial oxygenation.

The asphyxiated preterm model had perinatal acidosis as shown in Table 1, which improved significantly with DCCV (7.02 ± 0.08) compared to ECCV (6.96 ± 0.13). The difference in pH was statistically significant throughout the first 5 min of PPV ($p = 0.02$). The HR improved in both groups by 5 min—DCCV (180 ± 20 bpm) and ECCV (188 ± 30 bpm). The mean blood pressures in both groups by 5 min were similar (DCCV (40 ± 10 mmHg) and ECCV (44 ± 15 mmHg)).

3.1. Oxygenation

A higher percentage of lambs achieved preductal saturation targets in the DCCV group (75%) in the first 5 min compared to ECCV (60%). However, this result was not statistically significant (p-0.065). Preductal SpO_2 was significantly higher in the DCCV group compared to ECCV (p-0.01) (Figure 1).

The required oxygen concentration to achieve these target SpO_2 were significantly higher in the ECCV group compared to the DCCV group (Figure 2).

Oxygen load (OL)—as mentioned previously, OL was calculated using the tidal volume (TV) per kg in the first 5 min. The average TV in ECCV and DCCV were 6.0 ± 1.5 mL/kg and 6.0 ± 2.3 mL/kg, respectively. The OL with DCCV (520 (414–530) mLO_2/kg) was significantly lower compared to ECCV (775 (630–867) mLO_2/kg) ($p = 0.03$) as shown in Figure 3.

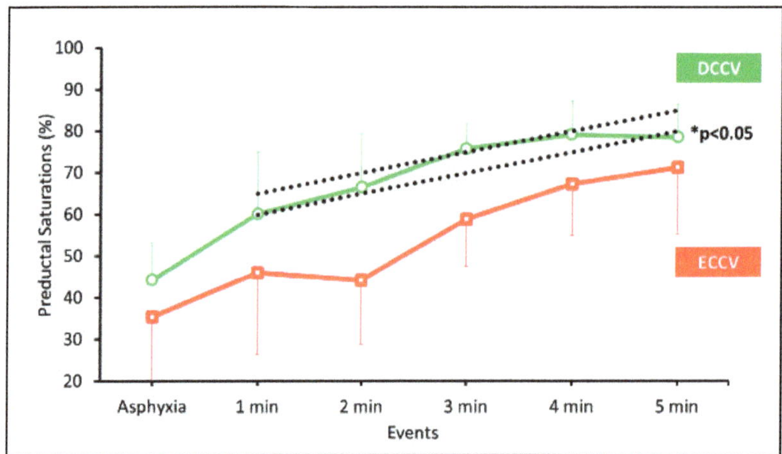

Figure 1. Preductal SpO_2 are shown on the y-axis and the events or duration of positive pressure ventilation (PPV) on the x-axis. The data are represented as average and standard deviation. The SpO_2 between ECCV (early cord clamping followed by ventilation) and DCCV (delayed cord clamping with ventilation) was significantly different (* $p < 0.05$ by ANOVA).

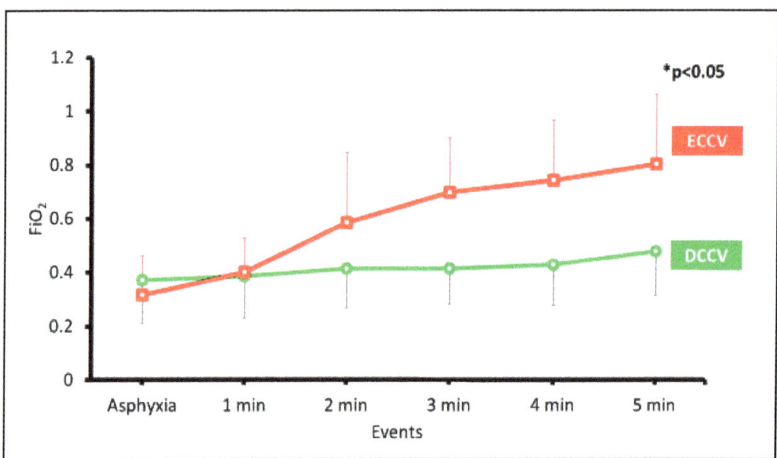

Figure 2. Fraction of inspired oxygen (FiO_2) is shown on the y-axis and the events or duration of PPV on the x-axis. The data are represented as average and standard deviation. The difference between ECCV and DCCV was significantly different (* $p < 0.05$ by ANOVA).

Arterial oxygenation (PaO_2)—despite the lower percentage of SpO_2 targets with ECCV, the PaO_2 was significantly higher (95 ± 65 mmHg) compared to DCCV (38 ± 9 mmHg, p-0.007) (Figure 4). The variability in arterial oxygenation with DCCV was minimal compared to ECCV, as shown by the standard deviations in Figure 4. The PaO_2/FiO_2 ratio at 5 min of PPV was 98 ± 50 in the DCCV group and 135 ± 87 mmHg in the ECCV group (p-0.4).

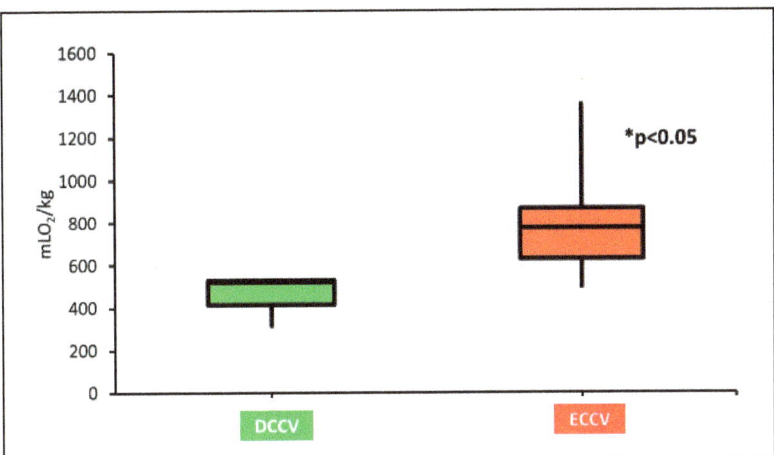

Figure 3. The oxygen load (OL) in milliliters of oxygen per kilogram is shown on the y-axis. The box and whiskers plot shows a significantly higher OL with ECCV compared to DCCV. OL in ECCV was significantly higher compared to DCCV (* $p < 0.05$ by Kruskal-Wallis test).

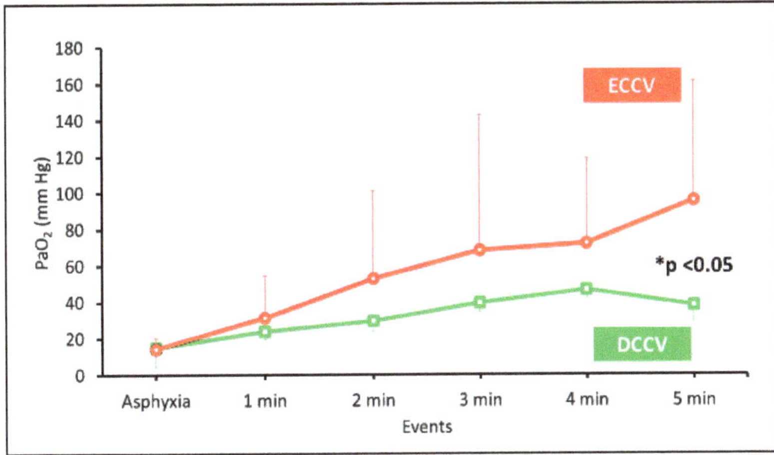

Figure 4. The PaO_2 in mm Hg is shown on the y-axis and the events or duration of PPV on the x-axis. The PaO_2 was significantly lower in DCCV (* $p < 0.05$ by ANOVA).

3.2. Ventilation

As mentioned previously, despite similar TV and ventilation rates in both groups in the first 5 min, the arterial carbon dioxide ($PaCO_2$) levels were significantly lower with DCCV compared to ECCV (Figure 5).

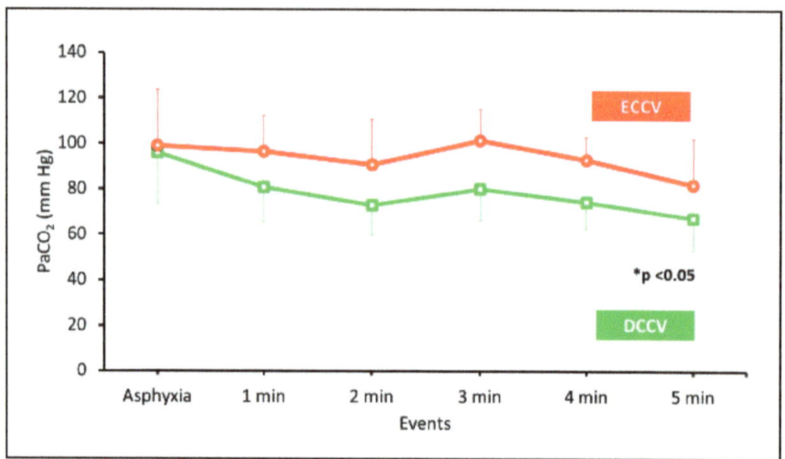

Figure 5. The arterial carbon dioxide ($PaCO_2$ in mmHg) is shown on the y-axis and the events on the x-axis. The $PaCO_2$ was significantly lower in DCCV compared to ECCV. (* $p < 0.05$ by ANOVA).

3.3. Hemodynamics

Pulmonary blood flow—the peak left pulmonary blood flows (PBF) were significantly higher in the DCCV group compared to ECCV (Figure 6).

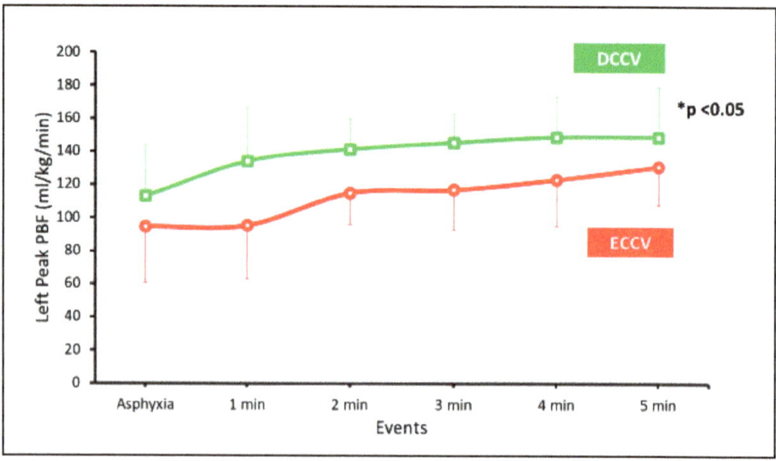

Figure 6. The left peak PBF is shown on the y-axis and the events on the x-axis. The PBF was significantly higher with DCCV compared to ECCV (* $p < 0.05$ by ANOVA).

Carotid blood flow—the peak left carotid blood flow (CBF) was not different between the two groups as shown in Figure 7.

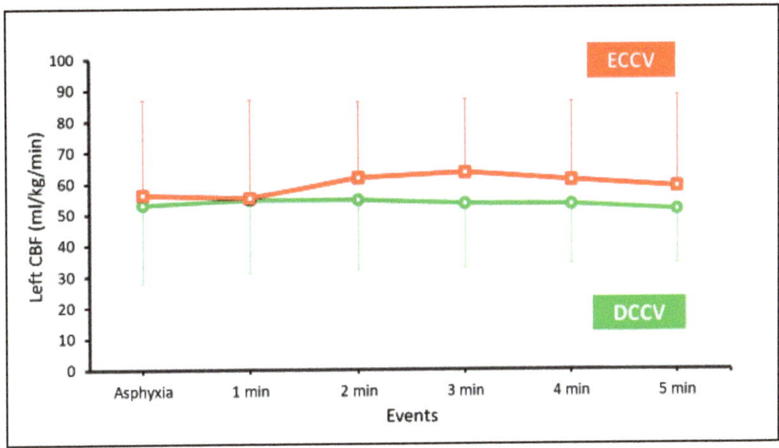

Figure 7. The left peak CBF is shown on the y-axis and the events or duration of PPV on the x-axis.

4. Discussion

In a depressed preterm neonate with HRs between 60–90 bpm, lower supplemental O_2, as currently recommended by NRP, may not achieve the pre-specified target SpO_2 or sustain pulmonary vasodilation. An alternative strategy is to ventilate with an intact cord and higher concentrations of supplemental O_2, especially in the setting of perinatal acidosis. Perinatal acidosis increases PVR. Low FiO_2 may not increase alveolar oxygen adequately to induce pulmonary vasodilation in preterm infants with high PVR. A combination of increased FiO_2 and resuscitation with an intact cord results in "transient alveolar hyperoxia" without systemic hyperoxia due to "buffering" of PaO_2 by umbilical venous return (Figures 4 and 8). Such "differential oxygenation" may be an effective concept for the resuscitation of depressed preterm infants that do not show spontaneous respiratory activity. The second advantage of resuscitation with an intact cord is "dual-site" gas exchange enabling CO_2 elimination in both the lungs and placenta.

In our pilot study, we tested our concept of "differential oxygenation" and "dual-site gas exchange" in a surfactant-deficient asphyxiated preterm lamb. We assessed the success of achieving target preductal saturation, gas exchange, and hemodynamics during ventilation with an intact cord as compared to the current standard of early cord clamping followed by resuscitation.

Arterial $PaCO_2$ levels were significantly lower in the DCCV group despite similar inflation pressures, tidal volumes, and ventilator rates (Figure 5). We speculate the contribution of placental gas exchange during resuscitation with an intact cord for this decrease. More efficient ventilation leads to earlier normalization of pH with DCCV. Early normalization of $PaCO_2$ increases pulmonary blood flow and avoids cerebral hyperemia.

The success in achieving the target preductal SpO_2 in asphyxiated preterm lambs was similar in DCCV (75%) compared to ECCV (60%) lambs, although DCCV lambs required significantly lower FiO_2. Previous clinical studies have shown improved SpO_2 in the first few minutes after birth with an intact cord compared to immediate cord clamping [16,18,22]. Recently, the preductal SpO_2 curves in spontaneous breathing term infants with an intact cord for a min were developed by Padilla-Sánchez et al. These curves show increased SpO_2 compared to immediate cord clamping, as shown in a study published by Dawson et al. [13].

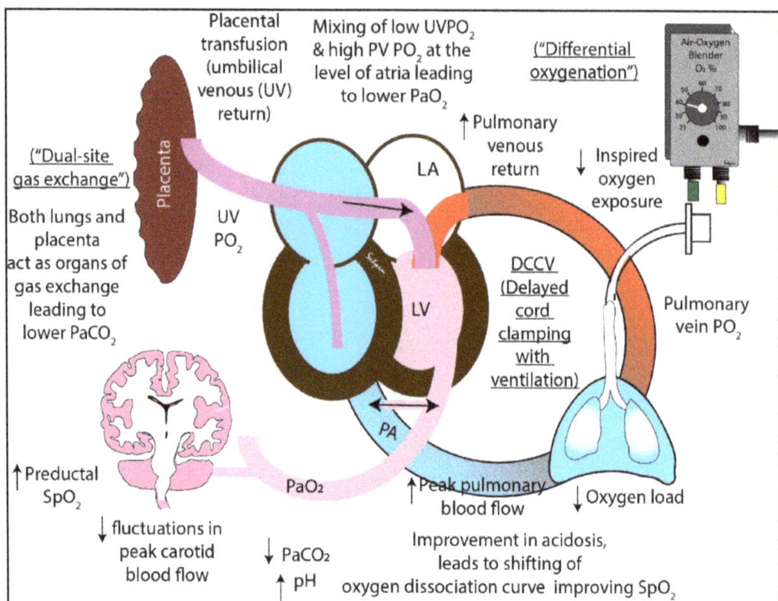

Figure 8. The benefits of delayed cord clamping and ventilation (DCCV) for 5 min in a lamb model of preterm asphyxia. With positive pressure ventilation and an intact cord, there was a mixing of lower umbilical vein oxygen tension (UVPO$_2$) with higher pulmonary venous oxygen tension (PVO$_2$) leading to overall systemic lower oxygen tension (PaO$_2$)—"differential oxygenation" with alveolar hyperoxia but systemic normoxia. With the placenta and lungs simultaneously acting as organs of gas exchange, the arterial carbon dioxide (PaCO$_2$) was lower ("dual-site gas exchange"). Copyright Satyan Lakshminrusimha.

Our study's striking feature was that the arterial oxygenation was much lower with decreased variability (as observed by lower standard deviations) in the DCCV group compared to the ECCV in the first 5 min. We speculate that the mixing of higher PO$_2$ pulmonary venous return with lower PO$_2$ in the umbilical venous return in the atrium, reduces systemic oxygenation as evidenced by lower PaO$_2$/FiO$_2$ ratios in the DCCV lambs. We speculate that, with a mix of PO$_2$ from the placenta and lungs, these term babies would have had lower PaO$_2$ compared to infants breathing with their umbilical cord cut despite higher SpO$_2$.

Despite lower PaO$_2$ in DCCV, the SpO$_2$ was significantly higher compared to ECCV. We speculate that the better SpO$_2$ reading in the DCCV lambs is due to two factors: better perfusion and prevention of a rightward shift in hemoglobin oxygen dissociation curve due to the rapid correction of acidosis. Asphyxia with combined respiratory and metabolic acidosis shifts the hemoglobin-oxygen dissociation curve leading to lower SpO$_2$ for a given PaO$_2$. We speculate that with better ventilation (lower PaCO$_2$) and higher pH in the DCCV group, SpO$_2$ values were higher despite lower PaO$_2$ levels in DCCV compared to ECCV [26]. By 5 min, the highest PaO$_2$ in DCCV was 38 $\pm$ 9 mmHg compared to ECCV, where it was 96 $\pm$ 65 mmHg. In a study, involving term neonates, Kapadia et al. have shown that perinatal acidemia and post-resuscitation hyperoxemia (defined as an initial PaO$_2$ of >100 mmHg) were associated with a higher incidence of hypoxic ischemic encephalopathy [27]. It is prudent to avoid high systemic PaO$_2$ and PaCO$_2$ values in asphyxiated preterm infants to limit cerebral hyperemia and oxidative reperfusion injury. Such injury can also predispose infants to intraventricular hemorrhage (IVH) in preterm neonates [28,29].

The oxygen exposure in the DCCV group was also much lower compared to the ECCV group. Hyperoxia in the delivery room is associated with an inflammatory response in the brain and the heart [30–34]. In a study involving an ovine model, hyperoxic resuscitation after fetal asphyxia led to the cerebral inflammatory response [34]. Secondary to the immature antioxidant response, oxidative injury in preterm infants can modify DNA methylation patterns, thus affecting gene expressions [35]. Lorente-Pozo et al. studied the effect of OL in preterm infants <32 weeks who were resuscitated with supplemental O_2 on DNA methylome [25]. The study concluded that OL during resuscitation altered DNA methylome that could potentially alter genes related to cell cycle progression, oxidative stress, and DNA repair [25]. In this study, the median OL during stabilization was 644 mLO_2/kg, and >500 mLO_2/kg could alter the methylation pattern. In our study, the OL in the first 5 min of resuscitation was 520 mLO_2/kg and was significantly lower than ECCV, which had an OL of 775 mLO_2/kg. In this asphyxiated model, the decreased OL observed in the DCCV group can decrease oxidative injury.

The significant improvement in peak left pulmonary blood flow observed in the DCCV was similar to a previous study by Bhatt et al. in a preterm non-asphyxiated ovine model [19]. The increase in PBF could possibly be secondary to stable hemodynamics, better pH with lower $PaCO_2$ in the DCCV group. Arterial oxygenation plays a great role in pulmonary vascular transition. Although the change point (PaO_2 value) for pulmonary vascular transition in an asphyxiated preterm neonate/model remains unknown, we have previously shown that in a non-asphyxiated preterm model, a PaO_2 of 31 ± 0.7 mmHg led to a drop in PVR [36]. In our study, we speculate that despite the lower PaO_2 observed in the arterial blood, higher alveolar PAO_2 helped overcome hypoxic pulmonary vasoconstriction and an improvement in pulmonary vascular transition in the DCCV group [26]. Custer et al. have shown that alveolar hypoxia could worsen hypoxic pulmonary vasoconstriction leading to a redistribution of pulmonary blood flow in a newborn ovine model [37]. Moreover, acidosis exacerbates hypoxic pulmonary vasoconstriction and better pH in DCCV could have ameliorated this effect, thus, leading to improved pulmonary vascular transition compared to ECCV.

Our study had some limitations. The data presented here are only for the first 5 min to compare the parameters while ventilating with and without an intact cord. We did not perform a sample size/power calculation for this pilot study. We did not collect markers of oxidative stress injury and used OL as a surrogate. The study was done in a controlled setting with multiple experienced personnel and may not be the case in real-life scenarios. Species differences do exist, but this asphyxiated preterm model with surfactant-deficient lungs has been widely used to study gas exchange and hemodynamics in the setting of placental transfusion. Since this was a pilot study and the recommended initial supplemental oxygen range by International Liaison Committee on Resuscitation is 30–60%, we chose random initial oxygen concentration with an average initial O_2 concentration within the specified range. The distribution was similar in both ECCV and DCCV groups as shown in Figure 2.

5. Conclusions

In this pilot study, in an asphyxiated preterm ovine model with perinatal metabolic acidosis, ventilation with an intact cord for 5 min (DCCV), decreased oxygen exposure, decreased oxygen load, with improved ventilation, while increasing peak pulmonary blood flow compared to immediate clamping of the cord and ventilation (ECCV). In the future, we intend to study the effect of DCCV with low (30–60%) and high (60–100%) oxygen exposure and its effect on oxidative injury and its impact on pulmonary and systemic hemodynamics. Clinical trials evaluating the resuscitation of extremely preterm infants with an intact cord at different concentrations of supplemental oxygen are warranted.

Author Contributions: Conceptualization, P.C. and S.L.; methodology, all authors.; software, P.C., S.G., J.H., C.K.; validation, P.C., S.G., J.H., N.B., C.K., L.N., J.N., V.A., M.B., A.M., M.R., S.L.; formal analysis, P.C., S.G., J.H., C.K.; writing—original draft preparation, P.C., S.L.; writing—review and editing, P.C., S.G., J.H., N.B., C.K., L.N., J.N., V.A., M.B., A.M., M.R., S.L.; funding acquisition, P.C., S.L. All authors have read and agreed to the published version of the manuscript.

Funding: This research was funded by NICHD, grant number R03HD096510 (PC), RO1 HD072929 (SL) and NHLBI-K12 HL138052 (PC).

Institutional Review Board Statement: The study was approved by the State University of New York at Buffalo, IACUC ID–PED10085N. All studies were conducted as per IACUC/ARRIVE guidelines.

Informed Consent Statement: Not applicable.

Conflicts of Interest: Satyan Lakshminrusimha is a member of the Neonatal Resuscitation Program Steering Committee of the American Academy of Pediatrics (AAP). The opinions expressed in this manuscript are the author's own and do not reflect the official position of the AAP. All other authors declare no conflict of interest. The funders had no role in the design of the study; in the collection, analyses, or interpretation of data, in the writing of the manuscript, or in the decision to publish the results.

References

1. American Academy of Pediatrics. *Textbook of Neonatal Resuscitation (NRP)*, 7th ed.; American Academy of Pediatrics: Elk Grove Village, IL, USA, 2016; p. 326.
2. Wyckoff, M.H.; Wyllie, J.; Aziz, K.; de Almeida, M.F.; Fabres, J.; Fawke, J.; Guinsburg, R.; Hosono, S.; Isayama, T.; Kapadia, V.S.; et al. Neonatal Life Support: 2020 International Consensus on Cardiopulmonary Resuscitation and Emergency Cardiovascular Care Science With Treatment Recommendations. *Circulation* **2020**, *142*, S185–S221. [CrossRef]
3. Wyckoff, M.H.; Wyllie, J.; Aziz, K.; de Almeida, M.F.; Fabres, J.W.; Fawke, J.; Guinsburg, R.; Hosono, S.; Isayama, T.; Kapadia, V.S.; et al. Neonatal Life Support 2020 International Consensus on Cardiopulmonary Resuscitation and Emergency Cardiovascular Care Science With Treatment Recommendations. *Resuscitation* **2020**, *156*, A156–A187. [CrossRef]
4. Welsford, M.; Nishiyama, C.; Shortt, C.; Weiner, G.; Roehr, C.C.; Isayama, T.; Dawson, J.A.; Wyckoff, M.H.; Rabi, Y. International Liaison Committee on Resuscitation Neonatal Life Support Task, F. Initial Oxygen Use for Preterm Newborn Resuscitation: A Systematic Review With Meta-analysis. *Pediatrics* **2019**, *143*. [CrossRef]
5. Oei, J.L.; Saugstad, O.D.; Lui, K.; Wright, I.M.; Smyth, J.P.; Craven, P.; Wang, Y.A.; McMullan, R.; Coates, E.; Ward, M.; et al. Targeted Oxygen in the Resuscitation of Preterm Infants, a Randomized Clinical Trial. *Pediatrics* **2017**, *139*, e20161452. [CrossRef]
6. Chandrasekharan, P.; Rawat, M.; Gugino, S.F.; Koenigsknecht, C.; Helman, J.; Nair, J.; Vali, P.; Lakshminrusimha, S. Effect of various inspired oxygen concentrations on pulmonary and systemic hemodynamics and oxygenation during resuscitation in a transitioning preterm model. *Pediatr. Res.* **2018**, *84*, 743–750. [CrossRef]
7. March of Dimes. Available online: https://www.marchofdimes.org/complications/premature-babies.aspx (accessed on 1 November 2020).
8. Chiruvolu, A.; George, R.; Stanzo, K.C.; Kindla, C.M.; Desai, S. Effects of Placental Transfusion on Late Preterm Infants Admitted to a Mother Baby Unit. *Am. J. Perinatol.* **2021**. [CrossRef]
9. Fogarty, M.; Osborn, D.A.; Askie, L.; Seidler, A.L.; Hunter, K.; Lui, K.; Simes, J.; Tarnow-Mordi, W. Delayed vs early umbilical cord clamping for preterm infants: A systematic review and meta-analysis. *Am. J. Obstet. Gynecol.* **2018**, *218*, 1–18. [CrossRef]
10. Katheria, A.; Poeltler, D.; Durham, J.; Steen, J.; Rich, W.; Arnell, K.; Maldonado, M.; Cousins, L.; Finer, N. Neonatal Resuscitation with an Intact Cord: A Randomized Clinical Trial. *J. Pediatr.* **2016**, *178*, 75–80.e73. [CrossRef]
11. Knol, R.; Brouwer, E.; van den Akker, T.; DeKoninck, P.; van Geloven, N.; Polglase, G.R.; Lopriore, E.; Herkert, E.; Reiss, I.K.M.; Hooper, S.B.; et al. Physiological-based cord clamping in very preterm infant -Randomised controlled trial on effectiveness of stabilisation. *Resuscitation* **2020**, *147*, 26–33. [CrossRef]
12. Mercer, J.S.; McGrath, M.M.; Hensman, A.; Silver, H.; Oh, W. Immediate and delayed cord clamping in infants born between 24 and 32 weeks: A pilot randomized controlled trial. *J. Perinatol.* **2003**, *23*, 466–472. [CrossRef]
13. Padilla-Sanchez, C.; Baixauli-Alacreu, S.; Canada-Martinez, A.J.; Solaz-Garcia, A.; Alemany-Anchel, M.J.; Vento, M. Delayed vs Immediate Cord Clamping Changes Oxygen Saturation and Heart Rate Patterns in the First Minutes after Birth. *J. Pediatr.* **2020**, *227*, 149–156.e141. [CrossRef]
14. Perlman, J.M.; Wyllie, J.; Kattwinkel, J.; Wyckoff, M.H.; Aziz, K.; Guinsburg, R.; Kim, H.S.; Liley, H.G.; Mildenhall, L.; Simon, W.M.; et al. Part 7: Neonatal Resuscitation: 2015 International Consensus on Cardiopulmonary Resuscitation and Emergency Cardiovascular Care Science With Treatment Recommendations. *Circulation* **2015**, *132*, S204–S241. [CrossRef]
15. Pratesi, S.; Montano, S.; Ghirardello, S.; Mosca, F.; Boni, L.; Tofani, L.; Dani, C. Placental Circulation Intact Trial (PCI-T)-Resuscitation with the Placental Circulation Intact vs. Cord Milking for Very Preterm Infants: A Feasibility Study. *Front. Pediatr.* **2018**, *6*, 364. [CrossRef]

16. Andersson, O.; Rana, N.; Ewald, U.; Malqvist, M.; Stripple, G.; Basnet, O.; Subedi, K.; Kc, A. Intact cord resuscitation versus early cord clamping in the treatment of depressed newborn infants during the first 10 minutes of birth (Nepcord III)—A randomized clinical trial. *Matern Health Neonatol. Perinatol.* **2019**, *5*, 15. [CrossRef]
17. Armanian, A.M.; Badiee, Z. Resuscitation of preterm newborns with low concentration oxygen versus high concentration oxygen. *J. Res. Pharm. Pract.* **2012**, *1*, 25–29. [CrossRef]
18. Bancalari, A.; Araneda, H.; Echeverria, P.; Marinovic, A.; Manriquez, C. Arterial oxygen saturation and heart rate in term newborn in the first hour after birth. *Rev. Chil. Pediatr.* **2019**, *90*, 384–391. [CrossRef]
19. Bhatt, S.; Alison, B.J.; Wallace, E.M.; Crossley, K.J.; Gill, A.W.; Kluckow, M.; te Pas, A.B.; Morley, C.J.; Polglase, G.R.; Hooper, S.B. Delaying cord clamping until ventilation onset improves cardiovascular function at birth in preterm lambs. *J. Physiol.* **2013**, *591*, 2113–2126. [CrossRef]
20. Brouwer, E.; Knol, R.; Vernooij, A.S.N.; van den Akker, T.; Vlasman, P.E.; Klumper, F.; DeKoninck, P.; Polglase, G.R.; Hooper, S.B.; Te Pas, A.B. Physiological-based cord clamping in preterm infants using a new purpose-built resuscitation table: A feasibility study. *Arch. Dis. Child Fetal. Neonatal. Ed.* **2019**, *104*, F396–F402. [CrossRef]
21. Hutchon, D.J. Ventilation before Umbilical Cord Clamping Improves Physiological Transition at Birth or "Umbilical Cord Clamping before Ventilation is Established Destabilizes Physiological Transition at Birth". *Front. Pediatr.* **2015**, *3*, 29. [CrossRef]
22. Kc, A.; Singhal, N.; Gautam, J.; Rana, N.; Andersson, O. Effect of early versus delayed cord clamping in neonate on heart rate, breathing and oxygen saturation during first 10 minutes of birth-randomized clinical trial. *Matern Health Neonatol. Perinatol.* **2019**, *5*, 7. [CrossRef]
23. Polglase, G.R.; Blank, D.A.; Barton, S.K.; Miller, S.L.; Stojanovska, V.; Kluckow, M.; Gill, A.W.; LaRosa, D.; Te Pas, A.B.; Hooper, S.B. Physiologically based cord clamping stabilises cardiac output and reduces cerebrovascular injury in asphyxiated near-term lambs. *Arch. Dis. Child Fetal. Neonatal. Ed.* **2018**, *103*, F530–F538. [CrossRef]
24. Polglase, G.R.; Dawson, J.A.; Kluckow, M.; Gill, A.W.; Davis, P.G.; Te Pas, A.B.; Crossley, K.J.; McDougall, A.; Wallace, E.M.; Hooper, S.B. Ventilation onset prior to umbilical cord clamping (physiological-based cord clamping) improves systemic and cerebral oxygenation in preterm lambs. *PLoS ONE* **2015**, *10*, e0117504. [CrossRef]
25. Lorente-Pozo, S.; Parra-Llorca, A.; Nunez-Ramiro, A.; Cernada, M.; Hervas, D.; Boronat, N.; Sandoval, J.; Vento, M. The Oxygen Load Supplied during Delivery Room Stabilization of Preterm Infants Modifies the DNA Methylation Profile. *J. Pediatr.* **2018**. [CrossRef]
26. Chandrasekharan, P.; Rawat, M.; Lakshminrusimha, S. How Do We Monitor Oxygenation during the Management of PPHN? Alveolar, Arterial, Mixed Venous Oxygen Tension or Peripheral Saturation? *Children* **2020**, *7*, 180. [CrossRef]
27. Kapadia, V.S.; Chalak, L.F.; DuPont, T.L.; Rollins, N.K.; Brion, L.P.; Wyckoff, M.H. Perinatal asphyxia with hyperoxemia within the first hour of life is associated with moderate to severe hypoxic-ischemic encephalopathy. *J. Pediatr.* **2013**, *163*, 949–954. [CrossRef]
28. Noori, S.; McCoy, M.; Anderson, M.P.; Ramji, F.; Seri, I. Changes in cardiac function and cerebral blood flow in relation to peri/intraventricular hemorrhage in extremely preterm infants. *J. Pediatr.* **2014**, *164*, 264–270.e3. [CrossRef] [PubMed]
29. Noori, S.; Seri, I. Hemodynamic antecedents of peri/intraventricular hemorrhage in very preterm neonates. *Semin. Fetal. Neonatal. Med.* **2015**, *20*, 232–237. [CrossRef] [PubMed]
30. Lakshminrusimha, S.; Russell, J.A.; Steinhorn, R.H.; Swartz, D.D.; Ryan, R.M.; Gugino, S.F.; Wynn, K.A.; Kumar, V.H.; Mathew, B.; Kirmani, K.; et al. Pulmonary hemodynamics in neonatal lambs resuscitated with 21%, 50%, and 100% oxygen. *Pediatr. Res.* **2007**, *62*, 313–318. [CrossRef] [PubMed]
31. Munkeby, B.H.; Borke, W.B.; Bjornland, K.; Sikkeland, L.I.; Borge, G.I.; Lomo, J.; Rivera, S.; Khrestchatisky, M.; Halvorsen, B.; Saugstad, O.D. Resuscitation of hypoxic piglets with 100% O2 increases pulmonary metalloproteinases and IL-8. *Pediatr. Res.* **2005**, *58*, 542–548. [CrossRef]
32. Wedgwood, S.; Steinhorn, R.H.; Lakshminrusimha, S. Optimal oxygenation and role of free radicals in PPHN. *Free Radic. Biol. Med.* **2019**, *142*, 97–106. [CrossRef] [PubMed]
33. Borke, W.B.; Munkeby, B.H.; Halvorsen, B.; Bjornland, K.; Tunheim, S.H.; Borge, G.I.; Thaulow, E.; Saugstad, O.D. Increased myocardial matrix metalloproteinases in hypoxic newborn pigs during resuscitation: Effects of oxygen and carbon dioxide. *Eur. J. Clin. Investig.* **2004**, *34*, 459–466. [CrossRef] [PubMed]
34. Markus, T.; Hansson, S.; Amer-Wahlin, I.; Hellstrom-Westas, L.; Saugstad, O.D.; Ley, D. Cerebral inflammatory response after fetal asphyxia and hyperoxic resuscitation in newborn sheep. *Pediatr. Res.* **2007**, *62*, 71–77. [CrossRef]
35. Hitchler, M.J.; Domann, F.E. An epigenetic perspective on the free radical theory of development. *Free Radic. Biol. Med.* **2007**, *43*, 1023–1036. [CrossRef] [PubMed]
36. Chandrasekharan, P.; Lakshminrusimha, S. Oxygen therapy in preterm infants with pulmonary hypertension. *Semin. Fetal. Neonatal. Med.* **2020**, *25*, 101070. [CrossRef]
37. Custer, J.R.; Hales, C.A. Influence of alveolar oxygen on pulmonary vasoconstriction in newborn lambs versus sheep. *Am. Rev. Respir. Dis.* **1985**, *132*, 326–331. [CrossRef] [PubMed]

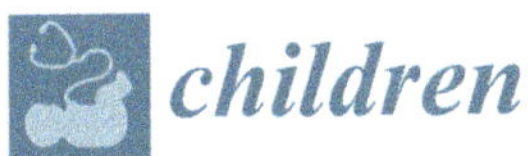 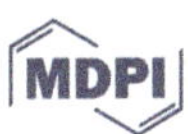

Article

Changes in Umbilico–Placental Circulation during Prolonged Intact Cord Resuscitation in a Lamb Model

Kévin Le Duc [1,2,*], Estelle Aubry [3], Sébastien Mur [2], Capucine Besengez [1], Charles Garabedian [1,4], Julien De Jonckheere [1,5], Laurent Storme [1,2] and Dyuti Sharma [1,3]

1. Univ. Lille, ULR2694 Metrics—Perinatal Environment and Health, F-59000 Lille, France; capucine.besengez@univ-lille.fr (C.B.); Charles.garabedian@chru-lille.fr (C.G.); julien.dejonckheere@chru-lille.fr (J.D.J.); laurent.storme@chru-lille.fr (L.S.); dyuti.sharma@chru-lille.fr (D.S.)
2. CHU Lille, Department of Neonatology, Jeanne de Flandre Hospital, F-59000 Lille, France; sebastien.mur@chru-lille.fr
3. CHU Lille, Department of Pediatric Surgery, Jeanne de Flandre Hospital, F-59000 Lille, France; estelle.aubry@chru-lille.fr
4. CHU Lille, Department of Obstetrics, Jeanne de Flandre Hospital, F-59000 Lille, France
5. INSERM CIC-IT 1403, CHU Lille, 59000 Lille, France
* Correspondence: kevin.leduc@chru-lille.fr; Tel.: +33-320-446-199

Abstract: Some previous studies reported a benefit to cardiopulmonary transition at birth when starting resuscitation maneuvers while the cord was still intact for a short period of time. However, the best timing for umbilical cord clamping in this condition is unknown. The aim of this study was to explore the duration of effective umbilico–placental circulation able to promote cardiorespiratory adaptation at birth during intact cord resuscitation. Umbilico–placental blood flow and vascular resistances were measured in an experimental neonatal lamb model. After a C-section delivery, the lambs were resuscitated ventilated for 1 h while the cord was intact. The maximum and mean umbilico–placental blood flow were respectively 230 ± 75 and 160 ± 12 mL·min^{-1} during the 1 h course of the experiment. However, umbilico–placental blood flow decreased and vascular resistance increased significantly 40 min after birth ($p < 0.05$). These results suggest that significant cardiorespiratory support can be provided by sustained placental circulation for at least 1 h during intact cord resuscitation.

Keywords: delayed cord clamping; intact cord resuscitation; umbilico–placental circulation

Citation: Le Duc, K.; Aubry, E.; Mur, S.; Besengez, C.; Garabedian, C.; De Jonckheere, J.; Storme, L.; Sharma, D. Changes in Umbilico–Placental Circulation during Prolonged Intact Cord Resuscitation in a Lamb Model. *Children* **2021**, *8*, 337. https://doi.org/10.3390/children8050337

Academic Editor: Simone Pratesi

Received: 31 March 2021
Accepted: 24 April 2021
Published: 26 April 2021

Publisher's Note: MDPI stays neutral with regard to jurisdictional claims in published maps and institutional affiliations.

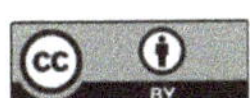

1. Introduction

Immediate umbilical cord clamping (ICC) affects cardiopulmonary transition at birth. ICC results in an increase in peripheral systemic vascular resistance and in a decrease in the inferior vena cava flow. Both an increase in afterload and a decrease in preload result in a decrease in systemic blood flow [1].

Conversely, delaying cord clamping between 30 and 180 s after birth increases the transfer of placental blood to the newborn, which increases the circulatory blood volume and prevents the risk of iron deficiency in infants 3 to 6 months old [2,3]. Numerous guidelines recommend delayed cord clamping (DCC) in the newborn infants who did not require immediate resuscitation in order to promote placenta to infant transfusion, although the timing of cord clamping is still debated [4–6].

Growing evidence suggests that DCC may promote cardiorespiratory adaptation in newborn infants who require resuscitation at birth. In an experimental study in newborn lambs, we highlighted that placental gas exchange can be sustained after birth, provided special care is taken to prevent compression or kinking of the umbilical cord [7]. Both arterial and venous umbilical blood flow were measured during DCC using Doppler ultrasound in uncomplicated term vaginal deliveries [8]. Venous and arterial umbilical flow were measured for longer than previously described, and this was continued in about half of the babies until the cord was clamped after 5 min [8]. We further showed the feasibility, safety, and effects of intact cord resuscitation in newborn infants with congenital diaphragmatic hernia [9]. Apgar scores were higher and plasma lactate concentrations were lower at 1 h after birth in the infants who were resuscitated, while the umbilical cord remained intact [9]. In this study, the cord was clamped once the baby was intubated and mechanically ventilated at around 7 min. Whether or not umbilico–placental flow can be prolonged any longer is still an open question.

Therefore, we hypothesize that umbilico–placental circulation can be sustained during intact cord resuscitation, provided the cord is secured carefully. To test the hypothesis, we continuously measured the umbilico–placental blood flow and resistance after birth during resuscitation in an experimental model of newborn lambs.

2. Materials and Methods

2.1. Experimental Model

All animal procedures and protocols used in this study (experimental research protocol n° 2017121218333678) received prior approval from the French Ministry of Agriculture (Ministère de l'Agriculture, de la Pêche et de l'Alimentation) before the study was carried out in the Department of Experimental Research at Lille University (animal experimentation agreement number D59-35010). Pregnant ewes of the Ile de France breed were hosted in individual pens starting a week before and throughout the procedure.

2.2. Surgical Procedure

At 138 ± 3 days gestation (term is about 142 days), under sterile conditions and general anesthesia (induction of anesthesia in the ewe with Xylazine–Sédaxylan®, 0.05 mg per kg and maintained with 2–5% isoflurane Aerane® in room air/oxygen following intubation) [10,11], the fetal lamb's left lower limb was exteriorized through a midline laparotomy and hysterotomy of the pregnant ewe.

After fetal analgesia (10 mg IM nalbuphine) and fetal local anesthesia (50 mg SC lidocaine hydrochloride), vascular polyvinyl chloride catheters (4Fr, Vygon® Ecouen, France) were advanced into the aorta after a skin incision in the groin area to measure the aortic pressure. The femoral arterial catheter was inserted to the 8 cm marker, corresponding to the bifurcation of the common umbilical artery of the abdominal aorta. The catheter in the left femoral vein was inserted up to 20 cm into the right atrium.

After a retroperitoneum section and after gentler, blunt dissection of the common umbilical artery at its root from the aorta, a flow transducer (size 6, Transonic System, Ithaca, New York, NY, USA) was placed around the vessel to measure umbilico–placental blood flow (Figure 1).

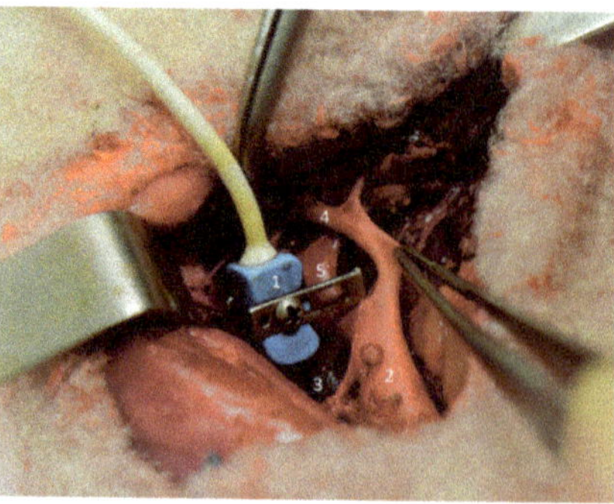

Figure 1. Setting up the probe doppler (**1**): aorta (**2**), vena cava (**3**), iliac artery (**4**), umbilical arteries (**5**).

Then, the lamb was exteriorized from the uterine cavity for exposure of the umbilical cord. In order to measure the umbilical vein pressure, a catheter (20 ga. Arrow) was introduced into one of the two umbilical veins at the base of the cord using the Seldinger technique.

Catheter patency was maintained by a bolus of heparinized saline, 10 UI/mL (Heparine CHOAY® 5000UI, Sanofi-aventis, Paris, France).

At the end of the experimental procedures, animals were euthanized using T61® (Tanax®, Intervet Beaucouzé, France: 3 mL/10 kg body weight for the ewe and 0.3 mL/kg for the lamb).

2.3. Experimental Design

In order to limit the heat loss and cooling of the lamb, a heat lamp was positioned above the table. The lamb was dried and placed on dry, warm clothes on a table above the ewe's hooves. Special care was taken to protect the cord from drying and to prevent stretching, kinking, or compressing of the cord.

During the entire resuscitation phase, the sedated pregnant ewe did not receive an injection of oxytocin in order to prevent placental delivery. The ewes are sedated with Isoflurane, and the newborn lambs are being resuscitated while the cord is intact: therefore, the lambs are anesthetized and sedated and do not breathe spontaneously. After pharyngeal suctioning, the lambs were intubated with a 4.5 mm cuffed endotracheal tube (Rüschelit®, Teleflex medical, Wayne, PA, USA). First, 20 s of sustained inflation at 35 cmH_2O was performed, and then the lambs were mechanically ventilated (Infant Star 950® ventilator, Covidien, Dublin, Ireland) in pressure controlled mode (PEEP 5 cmH_2O, Pmax 24 cmH_2O, FR 60/min, FiO_2 1) for one hour. After shaving the right foreleg and the right hind leg, preductal and postductal SPO_2 sensors continuously recorded blood oxygen saturation. Mechanical ventilation was adjusted to the target of 40–60 mmHg PCO_2. If the PCO_2 was greater than 60 mmHg, inspiratory pressure was increased by 5 cmH_2O. If PCO_2 was greater than 80 mmHg, inspiratory pressure was increased by 5 cmH_2O and respiratory rate was increased by 20 breaths per minute. The SpO_2 target was between 92 and 99%. FiO_2 was adapted every 5 min to reach the target. Rectal temperature was continuously recorded during resuscitation.

2.4. Hemodynamic and Biological Analysis

The flow transducer was connected to an internally calibrated flowmeter (T201, Transonic Systemes) for continuous measurement of umbilico–placental blood flow (Qup). The zero blood flow value was defined as the flow measured immediately before the beginning of systole. The aortic and the umbilical vein catheters were connected to a pressure transducer monitoring system (Merlin, Hewlett-Packard, Palo Alto, CA, USA). Heart rate (HR) was calculated using the phasic signal from the Qup. Umbilico–placental vascular resistance (Rup) was calculated as the difference between mean aortic pressure (Pao) and mean umbilical vein pressure (Pv) divided by mean umbilico–placental blood flow (Qup).

Blood samples (0.5 mL) from the aortic catheter were taken for blood gas analysis (ABL90 FLEX, Radiometer, Copenhagen, Denmark) 5 min before ventilation, at the beginning of the ventilation, and each 20 min after starting ventilation.

2.5. Statistical Analysis

The variables were collected just before and after starting mechanical ventilation. Each lamb served as his or her own control. All statistical analyses were conducted using SPSS Statistic version 24 (IBM corporation, Armonk, NY, USA). Continuous variables were mean ± standard deviation after checking for normal distribution of the data using the Shapiro–Wilk test. The non-parametric Friedman and Wilcoxon distribution-free test were used to assess the significance of differences in respiratory and hemodynamic measures between measurements.

3. Results

A total of five fetal lambs (mean weight: 3969 ± 488 g) were used for this experiment. One out of the five lambs was male. Blood gases during the experiment are displayed in Table 1. After 40 min of resuscitation, the blood gases improved with an increase in pH (7.1 to 7.3 at m40, $p < 0.05$) and a normalization of $PaCO_2$ (75 to 44 at M40, $p < 0.05$).

Table 1. Blood gas during the experiment.

Time	M0	M20	M40	M60
pH	7.1 ± 0.1	7.1 ± 0.2	7.2 ± 0.2	7.3 ± 0.1 *
PaO_2 (mmHg)	15 ± 4	126 ± 61 *	70 ± 29 *	68 ± 12 *
$PaCO_2$ (mmHg)	75 ± 17	62 ± 12	49 ± 11 *	44 ± 8 *
HCO_3 (mEq.L^{-1})	23 ± 8	20 ± 5	22 ± 6	23 ± 7

Values are means ± SD. PaO_2, arterial partial pressure of O_2; $PaCO_2$ arterial partial pressure of CO_2; HCO_3, bicarbonates. M0 represents the moment when mechanical ventilation was started; M60, the time at which the umbilical cord was clamped. * Significant difference accepted as $p \leq 0.05$.

Umbilical vein and arterial pressure did not change during the course of the experiment (Table 2).

Table 2. Respiratory and hemodynamic variables during the experiment.

Time	M-5	M0	M10	M20	M30	M40	M50	M60
HR (Beats/min)	147 ± 40	144 ± 35	133 ± 10	140 ± 20	132 ± 14	132 ± 13	140 ± 14	148 ± 14
PAo (mmHg)	43 ± 4	43 ± 8	48 ± 4	49 ± 4	47 ± 5	51 ± 7	53 ± 8	50 ± 6
Pv (mmHg)	7 ± 3	8 ± 2	8 ± 2	9 ± 2	9 ± 2	8 ± 2	8 ± 2	7 ± 2
Pre-ductal Spo2 (%)	80 ± 20	80 ± 20	98 ± 3	99 ± 2	97 ± 4	97 ± 3	98 ± 3	96 ± 2
Post-ductal Spo2 (%)	38 ± 23	38 ± 23	50 ± 32 *	90 ± 15 *	95 ± 6 *	93 ± 5 *	94 ± 3 *	95 ± 5 *
Qup (mL/min)	232 ± 38	234 ± 75	252 ± 107	214 ± 73	204 ± 98	186 ± 79	148 ± 33 *	158 ± 12 *
Rup (µW)	158 ± 10	151 ± 26	179 ± 66	205 ± 58	224 ± 104	262 ± 111	280 ± 106 *	299 ± 82 *

Values are means ± SD. HR, heart rate; PAo, mean aortic pressure; Pv, umbilical vein pressure; Pre-ductal Spo2, pre-ductal oxygen saturation; Post-ductal Spo2, post-ductal oxygen saturation; Qup, umbilico–placental blood flow; Rup, umbilico–placenta resistance. M0 represents the moment when mechanical ventilation was started; M60, the moment when the umbilical cord was clamped. * Significant difference accepted as $p \leq 0.05$.

Throughout resuscitation with an intact cord, a constant placental blood flow of 150 ± 22 mL·min^{-1} at M60 persisted with a statistically significant decrease from M40 compared to M0 (234 ± 75 to 186 ± 79 mL·min^{-1}, $p < 0.05$).

Placental vascular resistance gradually increased 1 h after birth, with no statistically significant difference between M0 and M40 (158 ± 10 to 262 ± 111 µW).

4. Discussion

Evidence suggests that starting resuscitation maneuvers while the umbilical cord is intact may promote cardiorespiratory adaptation at birth. However, the potential duration of placental circulation after birth is unknown. In the present study, changes in umbilico–placental circulation during intact cord resuscitation were assessed in experiments with fetal lambs. Although umbilico–placental blood flow was sustained until the end of the experiments at 60 min of resuscitation, umbilico–placental blow flow decreased and umbilico–placental vascular resistance increased steadily from 40 min onward. These results suggest that significant cardiorespiratory support can be provided by sustained placental circulation for at least 1 h during intact cord resuscitation.

International resuscitation guidelines currently recommend delaying cord clamping for 60 s in infants who do not need resuscitation, which is largely based on the concept of placenta to infant blood transfusion [12]. Controversies exist regarding the best timing of cord clamping in the newborn infants who need resuscitation. A previous study in newborn infants measured significant blood flow in both the umbilical artery and the umbilical vein for at least 5 min [8]. A previous study by Lefebvre et al. explored the feasibility and effectiveness of intact cord resuscitation in newborn infants with congenital diaphragmatic hernia. In that study, the cord was clamped by 7 min after birth. Apgar scores were significantly higher in the intact cord resuscitation group than in the immediate cord clamp group at 1 min and at 5 min [9]. In a spontaneous breathing lamb model, the cord was clamped at 20 min once the lamb was found to have established a stable breathing pattern [13]. In that study, umbilical blood flow was sustained until cord clamping, although it was transiently reduced during individual breaths.

To the best of our knowledge, our study is the first to explore the potential duration of umbilico–placental circulation after birth during intact cord resuscitation. The blood flow was measured at the root of the umbilical artery before its division into two umbilical arteries. This measure represents the blood flow circulating across the placenta and returning to the lamb via the umbilical vein. The driving force of the placental blood flow is the difference between the aortic pressure and the pressure measured at the distal extremity of the umbilical vein. We found that a maximum of about 250 mL/min of blood crosses the placenta after 10 min of intact cord resuscitation, which may represent 30% of the systemic blood flow of the lamb [14–16]. A steady increase of the umbilico–placental vascular resistance beginning 40 min after starting intact cord resuscitation explains the decrease in placental blood flow, as neither aortic nor umbilical vein pressures changed during the 1 h course of the experiment. We have shown that placental blood flow is stable up to 40 min after birth. During pregnancy, the placenta participates in the oxygenation and decarboxylation of the fetus. During delayed cord clamping resuscitation, we showed that PaO_2 promptly increased and $PaCO_2$ decreased. It would be interesting to study the evolution of placental O_2 uptake (placental VO_2) during delayed cord resuscitation. Our results indicate that effective cardiorespiratory support can be expected for a prolonged period of time during intact cord resuscitation in the conditions of our experiment.

Oxygen pressure into umbilical arterial blood during pregnancy is around 18 mmHg. In vitro studies on umbilical artery rings indicate that an increase in PO_2 induces an increase in the vascular tone, with a maximum contraction response observed at a PO_2 around 280 mmHg [17]. These results suggest that high PaO_2 during intact cord resuscitation may promote an increase in the umbilical vascular resistance and may contribute to a rapid drop of the umbilico–placental blood flow after birth. In our study, FiO_2 was adjusted to maintain a physiological SpO_2. The PaO_2 was around 60 mmHg during the study period. Our data indicate that an increase in PaO_2 within the normal range does not impair the umbilical circulation during intact cord resuscitation. Whether or not hyperoxemia may alter the umbilico–placental circulation remains an open question.

In routine clinical practice, oxytocin is infused just after birth for its uterotonic effects in order to prevent postpartum hemorrhage [18]. Oxytocin is known to induce vasoconstriction and increase significantly the uterine and umbilical artery flow resistance during uterine contractions [19]. Furthermore, oxytocin promotes placenta delivery. In our study, oxytocin was not infused at birth to the pregnant ewe after c-section to preserve umbilico–placental resistance. It is likely that oxytocin alters the course of the umbilico–placental circulation during intact cord resuscitation.

During the experiment and the intact cord resuscitation period, the pregnant ewes were anesthetized with isoflurane. Isoflurane has been reported to reduce the contraction of the uterine muscle. Indeed, isoflurane causes uterine relaxation through inhibition of the voltage-dependent calcium channels of the uterine smooth muscle cells [20]. Isoflurane may have delayed normal placental delivery and contributed to sustained placental circulation.

Previous studies showed that gas exchange can be sustained for up to 30 min during Ex utero Intrapartum Treatment (EXIT) procedure [21,22]. EXIT surgery is performed under general anesthesia to achieve uterine relaxation. The fetus is not delivered from the uterus: only the head, neck, and upper part of the thorax is exposed for the maintenance of the uterine volume, thus decreasing the likelihood of uterine contraction and placental abruption. EXIT may be indicated in case of high suspicion of fetal airway obstruction, such as cervical or oral tumors with a consequent high risk of severe fetal hypoxia or death of the newborn infant at birth. EXIT is a complex coordinated procedure that requires a multidisciplinary expert team, including pediatric surgeons, anesthesiologists, obstetricians, and neonatologists.

In the present study, the resuscitation maneuvers are started after birth while the cord is intact. Compared to EXIT, intact cord resuscitation can be used routinely and does not require a multidisciplinary and specialized team. To our knowledge, no study explored the change in umbilico–placental circulation after birth beyond 20 min during intact cord resuscitation.

Our study has limitations. Placenta in sheep (cotyledons) and humans (chorioallantoic) are different. The reproducibility of our physiopathological observations and therefore their extrapolation to the human newborn infants must be done with caution. The study was performed in normal lambs. Further study is required to assess the effects of prolonged intact cord resuscitation in an experimental model of impaired cardiorespiratory adaptation at birth. The present experimental study is a pre-requisite for further studies aiming at assessing the effectiveness of prolonged intact cord resuscitation in cases at high risk for abnormal cardiorespiratory adaptation at birth.

5. Conclusions

Our results indicate that effective umbilico–placental circulation can be sustained for up to one hour during intact cord resuscitation in the condition of our experiment including maternal isoflurane anesthesia and excluding oxytocin administration. Our study supports the hypothesis that the duration of intact cord resuscitation may be continued beyond 10 min in order to promote cardiorespiratory adaptation at birth. This information is interesting, because in situations with expected high perinatal mortality such as diaphragmatic hernia and severe hydrops, continuing intact cord resuscitation for up to 1 h could allow better adaptation to extrauterine life.

Author Contributions: Conceptualization, K.L.D., L.S., D.S., S.M., E.A., C.G.; methodology, K.L.D., L.S., D.S., S.M.; validation, K.L.D., L.S., D.S., C.G.; formal analysis, J.D.J. and K.L.D.; writing—original draft preparation, K.L.D.; writing—review and editing, K.L.D., L.S. and D.S.; supervision, L.S.; project administration funding acquisition, D.S., C.B. All authors have read and agreed to the published version of the manuscript.

Funding: This research was funded by the Rare Disease Foundation (Fondation Maladies Rares) (grant number# FONDATION_LAM-RD_201802).

Institutional Review Board Statement: The study was conducted according to the guidelines of the Declaration of Helsinki, and approved by the French Ministry of Agriculture (Ministère de l'Agriculture, de la Pêche et de l'Alimentation). Animal experimentation agreement number D5935010.

Informed Consent Statement: Not applicable.

Data Availability Statement: The data which we presented in the study are available from authors on request. The data are not publicly available due to privacy restrictions.

Acknowledgments: The authors would like to thank Thomas Hubert and Arnold Dive, Michel Pottier, and Martin Fourdrinier, animal caregivers of the DHURE Lille North of France, for their veterinary care and assistance for sheep anaesthesiology and surgery.

Conflicts of Interest: The authors declare no conflict of interest. The funders had no role in the design of the study; in the collection, analyses, or interpretation of data; in the writing of the manuscript, or in the decision to publish the results.

References

1. Crossley, K.J.; Allison, B.J.; Polglase, G.R.; Morley, C.J.; Davis, P.G.; Hooper, S.B. Dynamic Changes in the Direction of Blood Flow through the Ductus Arteriosus at Birth: Blood Flow through the Ductus Arteriosus at Birth. *J. Physiol.* **2009**, *587*, 4695–4704. [CrossRef] [PubMed]
2. McDonald, S.J.; Middleton, P. Effect of timing of umbilical cord clamping of term infants on maternal and neonatal outcomes. In *Cochrane Database of Systematic Reviews*; The Cochrane Collaboration, Ed.; John Wiley & Sons, Ltd.: Chichester, UK, 2008; p. CD004074.pub2.
3. Pratesi, S.; Montano, S.; Ghirardello, S.; Mosca, F.; Boni, L.; Tofani, L.; Dani, C. Placental Circulation Intact Trial (PCI-T)-Resuscitation With the Placental Circulation Intact vs. Cord Milking for Very Preterm Infants: A Feasibility Study. *Front. Pediatr.* **2018**, *6*, 364. [CrossRef] [PubMed]
4. Farrar, D.; Airey, R.; Law, G.R.; Tuffnell, D.; Cattle, B.; Duley, L. Measuring Placental Transfusion for Term Births: Weighing Babies with Cord Intact. *BJOG* **2011**, *118*, 70–75. [CrossRef] [PubMed]
5. Yao, A.C.; Wist, A.; Lind, J. The Blood Volume of the Newborn Infant Delivered by Caesarean Section. *Acta Paediatr. Scand.* **1967**, *56*, 585–592. [CrossRef] [PubMed]
6. Yao, A.C.; Lind, J. Blood Flow in the Umbilical Vessels during the Third Stage of Labor. *Biol. Neonate* **1974**, *25*, 186–193. [CrossRef] [PubMed]
7. Viard, R.; Tourneux, P.; Storme, L.; Girard, J.-M.; Betrouni, N.; Rousseau, J. Magnetic Resonance Imaging Spatial and Time Study of Lung Water Content in Newborn Lamb: Methods and Preliminary Results. *Invest. Radiol.* **2008**, *43*, 470–480. [CrossRef] [PubMed]
8. Boere, I.; Roest, A.A.W.; Wallace, E.; Ten Harkel, A.D.J.; Haak, M.C.; Morley, C.J.; Hooper, S.B.; Te Pas, A.B. Umbilical Blood Flow Patterns Directly after Birth before Delayed Cord Clamping. *Arch. Dis. Child. Fetal Neonatal Ed.* **2015**, *100*, F121–F125. [CrossRef] [PubMed]
9. Lefebvre, C.; Rakza, T.; Weslinck, N.; Vaast, P.; Houfflin-debarge, V.; Mur, S.; Storme, L. Feasibility and Safety of Intact Cord Resuscitation in Newborn Infants with Congenital Diaphragmatic Hernia (CDH). *Resuscitation* **2017**, *120*, 20–25. [CrossRef] [PubMed]
10. Houeijeh, A.; Aubry, E.; Coridon, H.; Montaigne, K.; Sfeir, R.; Deruelle, P.; Storme, L. Effects of N-3 Polyunsaturated Fatty Acids in the Fetal Pulmonary Circulation. *Crit. Care Med.* **2011**, *39*, 1431–1438. [CrossRef] [PubMed]
11. Houfflin-Debarge, V.; Sabbah-Briffaut, E.; Aubry, E.; Deruelle, P.; Alexandre, C.; Storme, L. Effects of Environmental Tobacco Smoke on the Pulmonary Circulation in the Ovine Fetus. *Am. J. Obstet. Gynecol.* **2011**, *204*, 450.e8–450.e14. [CrossRef] [PubMed]
12. World Health Organization. Nutrition for Health and Development. In *World Health Organization Guideline*; World Health Organization: Geneva, Switzerland, 2014; ISBN 978-92-4-150820-9.
13. Brouwer, E.; Te Pas, A.B.; Polglase, G.R.; McGillick, E.V.; Böhringer, S.; Crossley, K.J.; Rodgers, K.; Blank, D.; Yamaoka, S.; Gill, A.W.; et al. Effect of Spontaneous Breathing on Umbilical Venous Blood Flow and Placental Transfusion during Delayed Cord Clamping in Preterm Lambs. *Arch. Dis Child. Fetal Neonatal Ed.* **2020**, *105*, 26–32. [CrossRef] [PubMed]
14. Faber, J.J.; Green, T.J. Foetal Placental Blood Flow in the Lamb. *J. Physiol.* **1972**, *223*, 375–393. [CrossRef] [PubMed]
15. Kiserud, T.; Ebbing, C.; Kessler, J.; Rasmussen, S. Fetal Cardiac Output, Distribution to the Placenta and Impact of Placental Compromise. *Ultrasound Obstet. Gynecol.* **2006**, *28*, 126–136. [CrossRef] [PubMed]
16. Adamson, S.L.; Myatt, L.; Byrne, B.M.P. Regulation of Umbilical Blood Flow. In *Fetal and Neonatal Physiology*; Elsevier: Amsterdam, The Netherlands, 2011; pp. 827–837. ISBN 978-1-4160-3479-7.
17. McGrath, J.C.; MacLennan, S.J.; Mann, A.C.; Stuart-Smith, K.; Whittle, M.J. Contraction of Human Umbilical Artery, but Not Vein, by Oxygen. *J. Physiol.* **1986**, *380*, 513–519. [CrossRef] [PubMed]
18. Evensen, A.; Anderson, J.M.; Fontaine, P. Postpartum Hemorrhage: Prevention and Treatment. *Am. Fam. Physician* **2017**, *95*, 442–449. [PubMed]
19. Olofsson, P.; Thuring-Jönsson, A.; Marsál, K. Uterine and Umbilical Circulation during the Oxytocin Challenge Test. *Ultrasound Obstet. Gynecol.* **1996**, *8*, 247–251. [CrossRef] [PubMed]
20. Yamakage, M.; Tsujiguchi, N.; Chen, X.; Kamada, Y.; Namiki, A. Sevoflurane Inhibits Contraction of Uterine Smooth Muscle from Pregnant Rats Similarly to Halothane and Isoflurane. *Can. J. Anesth.* **2002**, *49*, 62–66. [CrossRef] [PubMed]
21. Novoa, R.H.; Quintana, W.; Castillo-Urquiaga, W.; Ventura, W. EXIT (Ex Utero Intrapartum Treatment) Surgery for the Management of Fetal Airway Obstruction: A Systematic Review of the Literature. *J. Pediatr. Surg.* **2020**, *55*, 1188–1195. [CrossRef] [PubMed]
22. Bouchard, S.; Johnson, M.P.; Flake, A.W.; Howell, L.J.; Myers, L.B.; Adzick, N.S.; Crombleholme, T.M. The EXIT Procedure: Experience and Outcome in 31 Cases. *J. Pediatr. Surg.* **2002**, *37*, 418–426. [CrossRef] [PubMed]

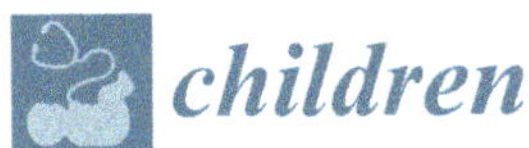

children

Article

Sustained Inflation Reduces Pulmonary Blood Flow during Resuscitation with an Intact Cord

Jayasree Nair [1],*, Lauren Davidson [1,2], Sylvia Gugino [1], Carmon Koenigsknecht [1], Justin Helman [1], Lori Nielsen [1], Deepika Sankaran [3], Vikash Agrawal [1,4], Praveen Chandrasekharan [1], Munmun Rawat [1], Sara K. Berkelhamer [1,5] and Satyan Lakshminrusimha [3]

1   Department of Pediatrics, University at Buffalo, Buffalo, NY 14203, USA;
    lauren.davidson26@gmail.com (L.D.); sfgugino@buffalo.edu (S.G.); carmonko@buffalo.edu (C.K.);
    jhelman@buffalo.edu (J.H.); lnielsen@buffalo.edu (L.N.); dragrawalmd@gmail.com (V.A.);
    pkchandr@buffalo.edu (P.C.); munmunra@buffalo.edu (M.R.); berkelsa@uw.edu (S.K.B.)
2   Buffalo Neonatology Associates, Sisters of Charity Hospital, Buffalo, NY 14214, USA
3   Department of Pediatrics, University of California at Davis, Davis, CA 95616, USA;
    dsankaran@ucdavis.edu (D.S.); slakshmi@ucdavis.edu (S.L.)
4   Department of Pediatrics, Loma Linda University, Loma Linda, CA 92350, USA
5   Department of Pediatrics, University of Washington, Seattle, WA 98195, USA
*   Correspondence: jnair@upa.chob.edu; Tel.: +1-7163-230-260

Abstract: The optimal timing of cord clamping in asphyxia is not known. Our aims were to determine the effect of ventilation (sustained inflation–SI vs. positive pressure ventilation–V) with early (ECC) or delayed cord clamping (DCC) in asphyxiated near-term lambs. We hypothesized that SI with DCC improves gas exchange and hemodynamics in near-term lambs with asphyxial bradycardia. A total of 28 lambs were asphyxiated to a mean blood pressure of 22 mmHg. Lambs were randomized based on the timing of cord clamping (ECC—immediate, DCC—60 s) and mode of initial ventilation into five groups: ECC + V, ECC + SI, DCC, DCC + V and DCC + SI. The magnitude of placental transfusion was assessed using biotinylated RBC. Though an asphyxial bradycardia model, 2–3 lambs in each group were arrested. There was no difference in primary outcomes, the time to reach baseline carotid blood flow (CBF), HR $\geq$ 100 bpm or MBP $\geq$ 40 mmHg. SI reduced pulmonary (PBF) and umbilical venous (UV) blood flow without affecting CBF or umbilical arterial blood flow. A significant reduction in PBF with SI persisted for a few minutes after birth. In our model of perinatal asphyxia, an initial SI breath increased airway pressure, and reduced PBF and UV return with an intact cord. Further clinical studies evaluating the timing of cord clamping and ventilation strategy in asphyxiated infants are warranted.

Keywords: sustained inflation; delayed cord clamping; placental transfusion; pulmonary blood flow; perinatal asphyxia

Citation: Nair, J.; Davidson, L.; Gugino, S.; Koenigsknecht, C.; Helman, J.; Nielsen, L.; Sankaran, D.; Agrawal, V.; Chandrasekharan, P.; Rawat, M.; et al. Sustained Inflation Reduces Pulmonary Blood Flow during Resuscitation with an Intact Cord. *Children* **2021**, *8*, 353. https://doi.org/10.3390/children8050353

Academic Editor: Simone Pratesi

Received: 7 April 2021
Accepted: 27 April 2021
Published: 29 April 2021

Publisher's Note: MDPI stays neutral with regard to jurisdictional claims in published maps and institutional affiliations.

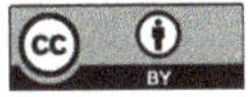

1. Introduction

Birth asphyxia affects 4 million newborn infants worldwide each year [1,2]. Appropriate resuscitative measures result in a substantial reduction in birth asphyxia-associated mortality and morbidity [3]. Establishing early and effective ventilation is key to successful neonatal resuscitation. Every 30 s delay in the initiation of ventilation increases the risk for early death and morbidity [4]. Sustained inflation (SI) may facilitate the early establishment of functional residual capacity (FRC). Revised European resuscitation guidelines recommend maintaining inflation pressure for 2–3 s for the first five inflations in apneic infants [5]. Minimal evidence exists for its use in term infants. A single SI immediately after birth improved the speed of circulatory recovery and lung compliance in the resuscitation of near-term asphyxiated lambs [6]. SI with continuous chest compressions is being evaluated as a resuscitation strategy in animal studies [7,8].

Available literature on SI is in neonatal/animal models with immediate or early cord clamping (ECC). ECC in asphyxia compromises both sources of LV preload (pulmonary venous (PV) return and umbilical venous (UV) return through the foramen ovale), resulting in decreased perfusion [9]. However, because of a lack of data demonstrating benefits and limitations of performing extensive resuscitation with an intact cord, delayed cord clamping (DCC) is currently not recommended, but is being evaluated in randomized controlled trials (e.g., SAVE NCT04070560). There is little information on resuscitation with SI and an intact cord. Our objectives were to determine the effect of ventilation (SI vs. positive pressure ventilation—PPV) with early or delayed cord clamping on resuscitation parameters in asphyxiated, bradycardic, near-term lambs. We hypothesized that SI with DCC would result in improved pulmonary and cerebral hemodynamics and enhanced gas exchange.

2. Materials and Methods

Surgical Protocol: The study was approved by the Institutional Animal Care and use committee (IACUC) at the University at Buffalo and the methods were consistent with the NIH guide for the care and use of laboratory animals (NIH Publications No. 8023, revised 1978) and in accordance with the ARRIVE guidelines. Time-dated ewes at 142–145d gestation (Term 147d) from May Family Enterprises (Buffalo Mills, PA, USA) were fasted overnight, then induced for anesthesia with intravenous diazepam and ketamine. Ewes were intubated and ventilated with 2–3% isoflurane. In total, 28 fetal lambs were partially exteriorized, intubated and drained of excess lung fluid to simulate the decrease in lung liquid with labor. ETT was occluded to prevent air exchange with gasping. Fetal lambs were instrumented [10] with catheters placed in the right carotid artery (CA) and jugular vein (JV) for blood pressure measurements and blood sampling. Flow probes (Transonic Systems Inc., Ithaca, NY, USA) were placed around the left CA, left pulmonary artery and one umbilical artery and vein. Preductal pulse oximetry was measured using a Nonin pulse oximeter sensor (EQUANOX™, Nonin Medical Inc, Plymouth, MN, USA). Asphyxia was induced by umbilical cord occlusion using a vascular occluder until the mean blood pressure (MBP) was less than or equal to 22 mmHg, when the cord was released, and lamb was exteriorized. In a prior study, the target MBP < 20 mmHg resulted in a need for extensive resuscitation and high mortality [6]. By initiating resuscitation at a MBP of 22 mmHg, we anticipated an adequate degree of asphyxia without extensive mortality or the need for advanced resuscitative efforts.

Randomization: Lambs were randomized prior to delivery to ECC (cord clamped immediately) and DCC (cord was clamped after 60 s). They were further randomized based on the timing of ventilation onset as well as the type of initial ventilation into five groups: ECC + V, ECC + SI, DCC, DCC + V and DCC + SI (Figure 1).

Resuscitation: A T-piece resuscitator was used for ventilation, with 21% O_2 at a rate of 40 breaths/min, an initial peak inflation pressure (PIP) of 35 cm H_2O and a peak end-expiratory pressure (PEEP) of 5 cm H_2O during the intervention period for all groups. The two SI groups—ECC + SI and DCC + SI—were resuscitated with an initial SI breath with a T-piece resuscitator with a PIP of 35 cm H_2O for 30 s. In the DCC group, ventilation was delayed until after the cord was clamped at 60 s. The intervention period was defined as the 30 s period when SI breath was delivered. In non-SI groups, the corresponding 30 s time period after the onset of resuscitation was taken as the intervention period. PIP was subsequently adjusted as needed to obtain an adequate chest rise, and PPV continued with 21% O_2 according to neonatal resuscitation guidelines [11] at a rate of 40–60 breaths/min in all groups. If lambs went into asystole, resuscitation was continued with CC and 100% oxygen [11]. Epinephrine (0.01–0.03 mg/kg/dose) was administered intravenously at 3 min for asystolic lambs. Inspired oxygen was titrated to maintain the recommended preductal SpO_2 [11]. Arterial blood gases were drawn at the initiation of resuscitation, then every minute for the first 5 min followed by every 5 min until the end of the study, and analyzed using a radiometer blood gas analyzer (ABL 800 FLEX, Copenhagen, Denmark).

Prespecified hemodynamic parameters were recorded for a period up to 30 min from birth, following which the lambs were euthanized using pentobarbital per approved lab protocols. Physiological parameters including heart rate (HR), systemic BP and vascular flows were continuously recorded using AcqKnowledge Acquisition and Analysis Software (BIOPAC systems, Goleta, CA, USA). An end-tidal carbon dioxide adapter was attached to the ETT and a Philips NM3 monitor (Respironics, Murrysville, PA, USA) was used to measure airway pressure.

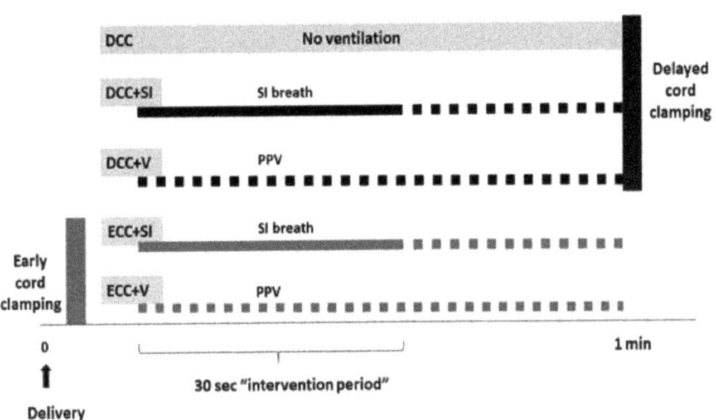

Figure 1. Study groups based on the timing of cord clamping and type of ventilation. DCC: Delayed cord clamping, ECC: Early cord clamping, SI: Sustained inflation, PPV: Positive pressure ventilation.

The magnitude of placental transfusion was assessed using biotinylated RBC to measure the red cell volume [12]. Next, 20 mL of maternal packed RBC was drawn a few days prior to the study and washed with a buffer solution three times. This was then divided into two groups; a low-density (LD) group of 12 ug/mL biotin and high-density (HD) group of 96 ug/mL biotin, both prepared with a target Hct of 50%. A baseline complete blood count (CBC) was drawn from the fetal lamb before injection. The low-density sample was infused into the lamb while still under maternal-fetal circulation, and samples were collected before and 10 min after injection to permit equilibration. This sample was used to measure the fetoplacental RBC volume. After delivery, the high-density biotin-labeled RBCs were injected to measure the newborn RBC volume. FICT-avidin (fluorescent marker) was added to the saved in vivo samples and measured with a flow cytometer. This labeled and counted the number of LD- and HD-labeled RBCs circulating in each sample to help determine the fetal vs. newborn total blood volume for each group studied.

The magnitude of placental transfusion was assessed between groups using the following equations.

(i)   RBC volume = Amount of biotinylated RBC injected ÷ concentration of biotinylated RBC in the sample after equilibration
(ii) Blood volume = RBC volume × 100 ÷ Hct
(iii) Residual placental volume = Fetoplacental blood volume—neonatal blood volume
(iv) Fraction of neonatal retained blood = Neonatal blood volume ÷ Fetoplacental blood volume.

Primary end-points: The primary end-point was the time to circulatory stabilization, defined as the time taken to reach the baseline carotid blood flow—CBF (prior to umbilical cord occlusion), stable HR ($\geq$100/min) and a MBP of $\geq$40 mmHg.

Secondary end-points: The secondary end-points included changes in systemic hemodynamics (CBF and MBP), left pulmonary blood flow (PBF) and umbilical arterial (UA) and venous (UV) flow changes during the 30 s intervention period between groups.

Statistical analysis and power calculation: Power and sample size calculations were based on a previous study of SI in asphyxiated near-term lambs [6], where the time to achieve circulatory stabilization within subject group was normally distributed with a standard deviation of 12 s. If the true difference in SI and PPV means was 25 s, we needed to study five subjects in each group to be able to reject the null hypothesis with a probability (power) of 0.8 and a Type I error probability of 0.05. Continuous variables were expressed as the mean and standard deviation (SD) and analyzed by ANOVA between groups with Fisher's post hoc test. Categorical variables were analyzed using the chi-square test with Fisher's exact test if appropriate. GraphPad Prism (San Diego, CA, USA) was used for statistical analysis. Statistical significance was defined as $p < 0.05$.

3. Results

Lambs were comparable in birth weight with similar baseline hemodynamic measurements that were obtained after instrumentation. The baseline UV flow was higher than the UA flow in most lambs. The extent of asphyxia was similar, as reflected by comparable pH and lactate levels (Table 1). Although intended as a model of bradycardia with perinatal asphyxia without cardiac arrest, 2–3 lambs in each group progressed to asystole similar to previously described studies in this model with cord occlusion [13].

Table 1. Baseline Characteristics.

	ECC + V ($n = 5$)	ECC + SI ($n = 6$)	DCC ($n = 5$)	DCC + V ($n = 5$)	DCC + SI ($n = 7$)
Weight (kg)	4.1 ± 0.8	4.3 ± 1	3.7 ± 0.8	3.6 ± 0.4	3.7 ± 0.4
Male	2	2	3	3	5
Multiple gestation	3	3	3	4	4
Incidence of arrest (epinephrine doses)	2 (1)	3 (2)	2 (2)	2 (2)	3 (1)
Baseline hemodynamics					
Left carotid blood flow (mL/kg/min)	28 ± 14	33 ± 10	24 ± 11	26 ± 11	33 ± 9
Mean systemic blood pressure (mmHg)	49	45	43	41	49
Mean umbilical venous blood flow (mL/kg/min)	29.8 ± 20	28.4 ± 17	34.2 ± 14.3	34.7 ± 11.1	49.2 ± 12.7
Mean umbilical arterial blood flow (mL/kg/min)	34.3 ± 29.6	22 ± 9	32.6 ± 9.8	31.4 ± 11.4	40.1 ± 18.5
Asphyxia blood gas					
pH	6.86 ± 0.1	6.88 ± 0.1	6.89 ± 0.0	6.88 ± 0.1	6.88 ± 0.1
pCO$_2$ (mm Hg)	111 ± 19	121 ± 11	123 ± 4	112 ± 34	119 ± 25
Lactate (mmol/L)	8.5 ± 2.5	9.0 ± 2.2	8.9 ± 2.3	9.8 ± 2.1	12.4 ± 2

3.1. Airway Pressure

As expected, the mean airway pressures in the SI groups, ECC + SI and DCC + SI, were significantly higher than in the PPV groups, ECC + V and DCC + V (Table 2), during the intervention period.

3.2. Primary Outcomes

No significant differences were noted among the five groups in time to reach baseline CBF, HR $\geq$ 100 bpm or MBP $\geq$ 40 mm Hg (Table 2).

3.3. Hemodynamics during Intervention Period

Among the DCC groups, the DCC + SI group had significantly decreased PBF compared to the DCC and DCC + V groups. MBP was comparable between groups (Table 2). Umbilical flows during the intervention period in all DCC groups were significantly lower compared to the baseline values prior to the onset of asphyxiation by cord compression. Significantly lower UV flow was seen during SI compared to DCC and DCC + V without any corresponding statistically significant differences in UA flow (Table 2).

Table 2. Primary outcomes and hemodynamic parameters during the intervention period.

	ECC + V (n = 5)	ECC + SI (n = 6)	DCC (n = 5)	DCC + V (n = 5)	DCC + SI (n = 7)
Primary Outcomes					
Time to reach baseline CBF (s)	115 ± 124	190 ± 83	295 ± 180	246 ± 246	207 ± 119
Time to HR > 100 bpm (s)	149 ± 101	151 ± 116	247 ± 161	243 ± 212	173 ± 126
Time to mean BP > 40 mmHg (s)	204 ± 189	217 ± 78	355 ± 181	281 ± 224	192 ± 107
During intervention					
Airway pressure (cmH$_2$O)	19.5 ± 5	37.7 ± 3	n/a	21.8 ± 6	34.6 ± 3 **
CBF (mean ± SD) mL/kg/min	12.1 ± 11.6	8.1 ± 10.8	4.9 ± 3.7	4.9 ± 2.7	6.7 ± 8.2
PBF (mean ± SD) mL/kg/min	2.1 ± 4.1	5.0 ± 6.7	3.6 ± 4.4	6.6 ± 6.4	1.3 ± 3.1 *
UV flow (mean ± SD) mL/kg/min	n/a	n/a	4.5 ± 3.4	2.9 ± 2.2	1.6 ± 3.6 *
UA flow (mean ± SD) mL/kg/min	n/a	n/a	3.1 ± 2.5	0.7 ± 1.6	1.3 ± 3.4
Mean BP (mean ± SD) mmHg	25 ± 13	21 ± 4	25 ± 6	21 ± 7	20 ± 9

Values are presented as mean ± SD; * $p < 0.05$ by Kruskal–Wallis one-way analysis of variance between DCC groups; ** $p < 0.005$ by Kruskal–Wallis one-way analysis of variance between groups.

3.4. Post Resuscitation Hemodynamics

CBF decreased during asphyxia and increased after birth in all groups (Figure 2a), reaching baseline values by 5 min. No statistically significant differences in CBF patterns were noted among the five individual groups. However, ECC + V and ECC + SI appeared to result in a rebound of cerebral blood flow above baseline, while DCC (with and without ventilation) resulted in a steady increase back to baseline values without overshoot. PBF (Figure 2b) in all lambs increased after birth; however, at 1–3 min, the PPV groups (ECC + V and DCC + V) demonstrated a trend towards higher PBF, compared to the SI groups (ECC + SI and DCC + SI). MBP and SBP (Figure 2c,d) were similar in the 30 min period after birth, with figures depicting the first 10 min.

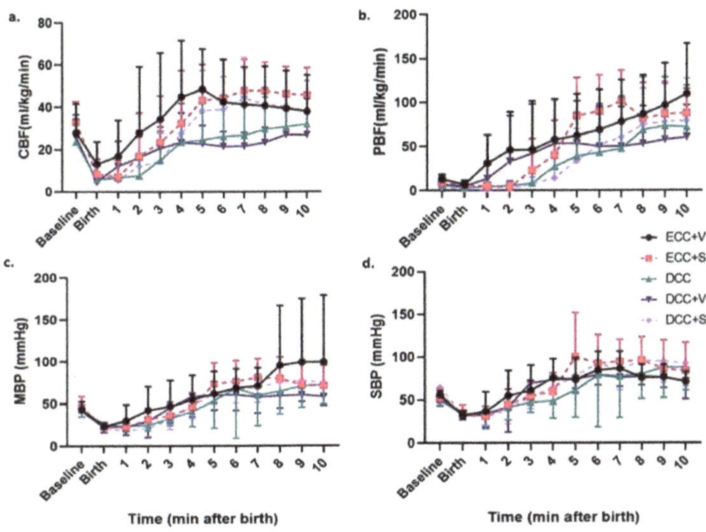

Figure 2. Post resuscitation hemodynamics in the first 10 min after birth in the five study groups: (**a**) carotid blood flow, (**b**) pulmonary blood flow, (**c**) mean blood pressure and (**d**) systolic blood pressure in all five study groups, with dashed lines reflecting the SI groups. Data are represented as mean ± SD. Black circle: ECC + V (n = 5), pink square dashed: ECC + SI (n = 6), green triangle: DCC (n = 5), purple triangle: DCC + V (n = 5), purple diamond dashed: DCC + SI (n = 7).

3.5. Gas Exchange and Lactate

Arterial pH, pCO_2, pO_2 and lactate were similar between groups at 2, 5 and 10 min, as were PaO_2/FiO_2 (P/F) ratios at 2 and 5 min. However, at 10 min, P/F ratios were significantly higher in the DCC + SI group along with a lower $PaCO_2$. Among the DCC groups, the required FiO_2 trended lower, and the P/F ratio was significantly higher in the DCC + SI group (Table 3).

Table 3. Gas exchange parameters.

	ECC + V (*n* = 5)	ECC + SI (*n* = 6)	DCC (*n* = 5)	DCC + V (*n* = 5)	DCC + SI (*n* = 6)
		Blood gas parameters at 2 min			
pH	6.9 ± 0.1	6.9 ± 0.1	6.9 ± 0.1	7.0 ± 0.2	6.9 ± 0.1
pCO_2 (mmHg)	107 ± 16	110 ± 14	130 ± 24	87 ± 24	92 ± 26
pO_2 (mmHg)	29 ± 24	27 ± 6	22 ± 14	29 ± 11	20 ± 8
FiO_2	0.5 ± 0.4	0.8 ± 0.3	0.5 ± 0.3	0.5 ± 0.4	0.8 ± 0.4
P/F ratio	106 ± 133	41 ± 24	51 ± 38	79 ± 65	39 ± 38
Lactate (mmol/L)	8.3 ± 1.8	8.7 ± 1.5	10.2 ± 2.4	8.9 ± 1.5	11.7 ± 2.5
		Blood gas parameters at 5 min			
pH	6.9 ± 0.2	6.9 ± 0.1	6.9 ± 0.1	6.9 ± 0.2	7 ± 0.2
pCO_2 (mmHg)	102 ± 27	95 ± 11	99 ± 39	90 ± 42	66 ± 36
pO_2 (mmHg)	61 ± 51	85 ± 50	37 ± 31	46 ± 30	45 ± 17
FiO_2	0.6 ± 0.4	0.7 ± 0.3	0.6 ± 0.3	0.4 ± 0.2	0.5 ± 0.4
P/F ratio	126 ± 132	138 ± 60	93 ± 106	149 ± 110	127 ± 113
Lactate (mmol/L)	8.9 ± 2.3	8.8 ± 1.9	9.4 ± 3.4	9.8 ± 3.8	11.2 ± 3
		Blood gas parameters at 10 min			
pH	7.0 ± 0.2	6.9 ± 0.1	6.9 ± 0.1	6.9 ± 0.2	7.0 ± 0.1
pCO_2 (mmHg)	81 ± 15	82 ± 27	83 ± 39	73 ± 34	44 ± 15 *
pO_2 (mmHg)	82 ± 36	106 ± 68	52 ± 30	76 ± 49	134 ± 80
FiO_2	0.5 ± 0.3	0.5 ± 0.3	0.8 ± 0.4	0.7 ± 0.4	0.3 ± 0.1
P/F ratio	180 ± 72	227 ± 165	98 ± 83	165 ± 156	400 ± 151 *#
Lactate (mmol/L)	8.5 ± 2.6	8 ± 2.1	10 ± 3.7	9.1 ± 2.5	11.8 ± 3.3

* $p < 0.05$ by Kruskal–Wallis test of variance in all groups; # $p < 0.02$ Kruskal–Wallis test of variance in DCC groups.

3.6. Magnitude of Placental Transfusion

Residual placental volume and newborn blood volume were similar between the ECC and DCC groups (Table 4). Speculating that placental transfusion was interrupted during arrest, we performed a subgroup analysis of non-arrested lambs. The DCC lambs had a significantly higher fraction of fetoplacental volume and a decreased residual placental volume compared to the ECC lambs (Table 4).

Table 4. Measurement of blood volume and placental transfusion.

A. All Lambs	ECC (*n* = 9)	DCC (*n* = 10)
Fetoplacental blood volume (mL/kg)	82 ± 20	76 ± 18
Newborn blood volume (mL/kg)	61 ± 14	60 ± 17
Residual placental blood volume (mL/kg)	21 ± 15	16 ± 13
Fraction of fetoplacental volume in newborn	0.76 ± 0.1	0.8 ± 0.2
B. Non-arrested	**ECC (*n* = 5)**	**DCC (*n* = 7)**
Fetoplacental blood volume (mL/kg)	92 ± 18	74 ± 19
Newborn blood volume (mL/kg)	58 ± 13	58 ± 12
Residual placental blood volume (mL/kg)	35 ± 8	16 ± 14 *
Fraction of fetoplacental volume in newborn	0.65 ± 0.1	0.84 ± 0.2 *

Values are presented as mean $\pm$ SD * $p < 0.05$ by Mann–Whitney U test vs. ECC.

3.7. Mode of Ventilation

Comparing SI (ECC + SI and DCC + SI) vs. PPV (ECC + V and DCC + V), the CBF patterns were not different (Figure 3a); however, the SI significantly reduced PBF in the first 4 min after birth (Figure 3b). MBP and SBP were similar with PPV or SI (Figure 3c,d).

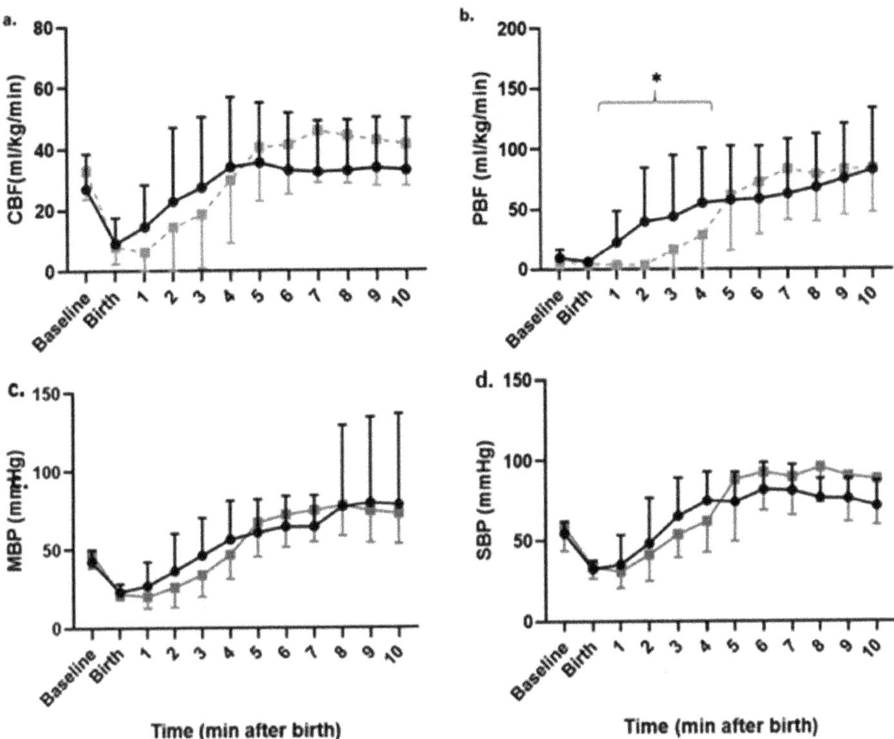

Figure 3. Post resuscitation hemodynamics in the first 10 min after birth in ventilation groups—effect of sustained inflation (gray squares, N = 13) is compared to positive pressure ventilation (Black circles, N = 10): (**a**) carotid blood (CBF), (**b**) pulmonary blood flow (PBF), (**c**) mean blood pressure (MBP) and (**d**) systolic blood pressure (SBP). Data are represented as mean $\pm$ SD. * $p < 0.01$ by repeated measures ANOVA.

3.8. Timing of Cord Clamping

DCC reduced the CBF overshoot that was noted with ECC during the post resuscitation period (Figure 4a). Both groups had similar PBF, MBP and SBP post resuscitation (Figure 4b–d).

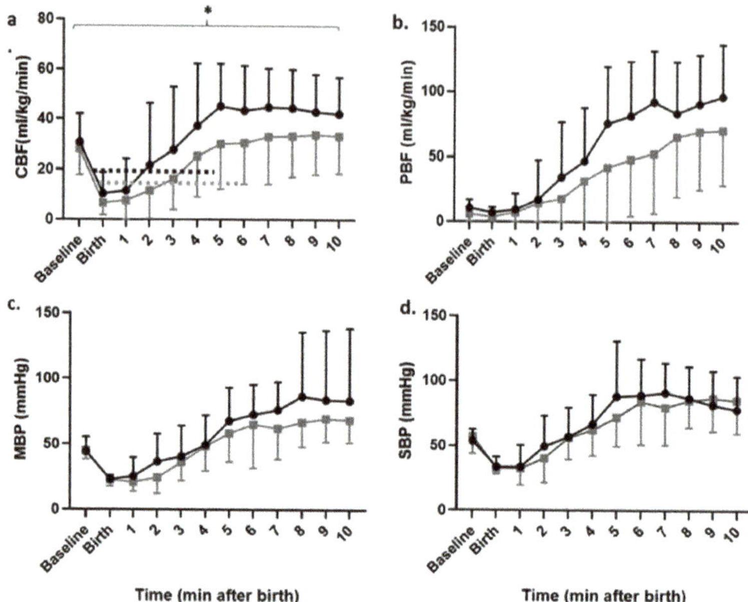

Figure 4. Post resuscitation hemodynamics in the first 10 min after birth based on the timing of cord clamping: (**a**) carotid blood flow, (**b**) pulmonary blood, (**c**) mean blood pressure and (**d**) systolic blood pressure. Data are represented as mean ± SD. * $p < 0.05$ repeated measures ANOVA. Black circles: ECC. Grey squares: DCC.

4. Discussion

In animal models and infants without asphyxia or with mild/moderate compromise, the benefits of physiological cord clamping (DCC after ventilation onset) are well established [9,14]. In our study, we compared DCC using two modes of ventilation, SI and PPV, which we compared to DCC without ventilation and ECC with immediate ventilation (current standard) in severely asphyxiated lambs. Few studies have evaluated DCC in a non-ventilated asphyxiated animal model. Delayed cord clamping for 60 s with ventilation mitigated post resuscitation cerebral hyperemia, but did not offer other substantial hemodynamic advantages. SI transiently decreased pulmonary perfusion, but led to a better gas exchange by 10 min when used in conjunction with DCC (Figure 5).

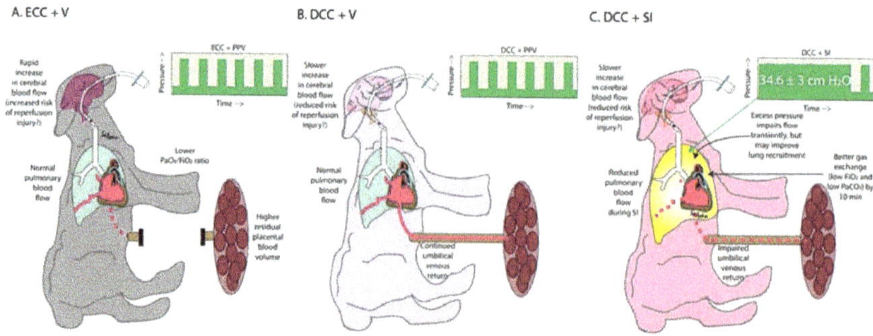

Figure 5. Summary: effects of (**A**) ECC + V—current practice, (**B**) DCC + V and (**C**) DCC + SI in our model of ovine asphyxia induced by cord occlusion.

SI as an initial ventilation strategy for lung recruitment has shown some benefits. A two-fold increase in inflation volume and FRC was described with SI in nine term asphyxiated newborns [15]. SI reduced the need for mechanical ventilation at 72 h [16] in preterm infants. Recently, the well-designed multicenter, randomized, SAIL trial evaluating SI in extremely preterm infants at birth was terminated early with infants in the SI group demonstrating increased early mortality [17], without any clear etiology. Interestingly, 15–20% of infants in both arms underwent 30 s DCC prior to SI, though their outcomes were not reported separately. A unique feature of our study is the evaluation of SI in combination with intact cord resuscitation. Contrary to our hypothesis, we could not demonstrate improved systemic or pulmonary hemodynamic outcomes with SI and DCC in an asphyxiated model. In fact, we report deleterious effects of SI on reducing PBF and UV flow, possibly due to an effect on intrathoracic pressure and/or diaphragmatic excursion [18] with an intact cord during the first few minutes after birth. However, these deleterious effects that we observed with a high pressure of 34.6 $\pm$ 3 cm H_2O with SI may not be seen with lower pressures in a non-asphyxiated model, with or without an intact cord.

Several different time periods and inflation pressures were evaluated in SI. We chose a 30 s SI breath with a peak inflating pressure (PIP) of ~35 cm H_2O and PEEP of 5 cm H_2O on the basis of prior studies in a similar model. Klingenberg et al. compared five 3 s inflations or a single 30 s inflation in resuscitation of near-term asphyxiated lambs with subsequent ventilation using inflations at 0.5 s at 60/min for all groups [6]. They noted earlier cardiovascular recovery (time taken to achieve a HR > 120/min) by almost 60 s in the single 30 s sustained inflation group compared to the no SI groups. We could not demonstrate a similar benefit to SI with either early or delayed cord clamping in our study; however, the incidence of cardiac arrest in our model complicated the analysis of this data.

While no differences in gas exchange were noted at 2 and 5 min, we demonstrated differences at 10 min (Table 3). We suspect that SI resulted in better recruitment of the lung establishing FRC, resulting in higher PaO_2 values. In addition, a combination of SI and DCC enabled "dual-ventilation" during the first 5 min, leading to normocapnia. Hypercapnia is known to enhance V/Q mismatch [19]. We speculate that lambs in the DCC + SI arm achieved a higher P/F ratio due to better alveolar recruitment and V/Q matching secondary to normocapnia (Table 3).

The interplay between different modes of ventilation and timing of cord clamping has not been evaluated before and is a strength of our study. There is insufficient evidence for or against DCC in infants requiring resuscitation [11]. Currently, most information on intact cord resuscitation in asphyxia comes from translational ovine models similar to our current study. DCC for 15 min restored cardiac output and oxygenation and mitigated post-asphyxial rebound hypertension after resuscitation in a non-arrest ovine model of perinatal asphyxia induced by maternal iliac artery ligation [13]. In lambs with asphyxial arrest, DCC for 10 min caused significant reductions in post-asphyxial rebound hypertension, cerebral blood flow and oxygenation [20]. These studies indicate improved hemodynamics with a longer DCC duration, and along with a difference in methodology of induced asphyxia (cord occlusion vs. maternal iliac artery ligation), may explain lack of sustained benefits in our study. With a clinically feasible and widely adapted shorter duration of a DCC of 60 s, we demonstrated the mitigation of post-asphyxial hyperemia in our model.

DCC is a reasonable option for term and preterm deliveries that do not require resuscitation. The negative intrathoracic pressure generated by a vigorous, crying neonate potentially assists placental transfusion [21], estimated at 20–40 mL/kg [22], and increases oxygen delivery by increasing arterial oxygen content and cardiac output [23]. However, PPV does not appear to enhance placental transfusion [24]. It is also unclear if placental transfusion occurs in cord occlusion-induced perinatal asphyxia, especially in infants are born via c-section. In our study, including all available lambs, we were unable to demonstrate any advantage to neonatal blood volume in lambs with delayed cord clamping, with and without ventilation. However, asphyxial arrest causes cessation of cord blood transfer. The non-arrested subgroup analysis showed reduced residual placental blood volume with delayed cord clamping, suggesting that placental transfusion does occur in this cohort.

We acknowledge several limitations of our study including obvious species differences. The use of maternal general anesthesia, fetal instrumentation and cesarean section could influence the results. However, these variables were common to all groups and between-group differences in results can be at least partly attributable to the randomized intervention. Unanticipated arrest was the biggest drawback of our model. As arrest occurred subsequent to the intervention period, we included them as an intent-to-treat analysis. The interventions may have contributed to progressive asphyxia and asystole. CC and epinephrine could affect post resuscitation hemodynamics, leading to large variation in results. Analyzing primary outcomes in the non-arrest subgroup was difficult due to small numbers, and these subgroup results are reported in the Supplementary Material (Table S1), where the current practice (ECC + V) resulted in a rapid return to baseline CBF. However, our unique translational model addresses important unanswered questions, with this study demonstrating complex interactions between ventilation techniques and cord clamp timing.

5. Conclusions

We conclude that higher airway pressures delivered by a 30 s SI breath in near-term asphyxiated lambs with DCC reduced both UV and PBF without affecting UA or CBF. A significant reduction in PBF with SI persists in the first few minutes after birth. We speculate that reduced PBF with SI may lead to delayed pulmonary vascular transition in this asphyxiated newborn model, already at increased risk for pulmonary hypertension/respiratory failure. However, DCC + SI resulted in lower CO_2 and a higher PaO_2/FiO_2 ratio. On the basis of our findings, we suggest that SI as a ventilation strategy, especially in combination with DCC, should be used with caution in asphyxia. Our findings reinforce the need for randomized clinical trials to evaluate optimal cord management and ventilation strategies in asphyxiated newborns.

Supplementary Materials: The following are available online at https://www.mdpi.com/article/10.3390/children8050353/s1, Table S1: Subgroup without Arrest—Primary Outcomes.

Author Contributions: Conceptualization, J.N. and S.L.; methodology and acquisition of data J.N., L.D., S.G., C.K., J.H., L.N., S.K.B., D.S., V.A., P.C. and M.R.; data curation, C.K., J.H., S.G. and L.N.; writing—original draft preparation, J.N.; writing—review and editing, J.N. and S.L.; supervision, S.L.; project administration, J.N.; funding acquisition, J.N. All authors have read and agreed to the published version of the manuscript.

Funding: This work was supported by the National Institutes of Health—Eunice Kennedy Shriver National Institute of Child Health and Human Development, 1 Center, Bethesda, MD 20892 1 R03 HD086531-01 (J.N.) and American Academy of Pediatrics, Itasca, IL, 60143 Neonatal Resuscitation Program Research Grant 2017 (J.N.).

Institutional Review Board Statement: The study was approved by the Institutional Animal Care Committee (IACUC) at the University at Buffalo (Protocol PED10085N, IACUC ID AR202000013) and methods were consistent with the National Institutes of Health guide for the care and use of laboratory animals (NIH Publications No. 8023, revised 1978).

Informed Consent Statement: Not applicable.

Data Availability Statement: The data presented in this study are available in this article.

Conflicts of Interest: The funders had no role in the design of the study; in the collection, analyses, or interpretation of data; in the writing of the manuscript, or in the decision to publish the results.

References

1. Nair, J.; Kumar, V.H.S. Current and emerging therapies in the management of hypoxic ischemic encephalopathy in neonates. *Children* **2018**, *5*, 99. [CrossRef] [PubMed]
2. Saugstad, O.D. Reducing global neonatal mortality is possible. *Neonatology* **2011**, *99*, 250–257. [CrossRef]
3. Vento, M.; Saugstad, O.D. Resuscitation of the term and preterm infant. *Semin. Fet. Neonatal Med.* **2010**, *15*, 216–222. [CrossRef]
4. Ersdal, H.L.; Mduma, E.; Svensen, E.; Perlman, J.M. Early initiation of basic resuscitation interventions including face mask ventilation may reduce birth asphyxia related mortality in low-income countries: A prospective descriptive observational study. *Resuscitation* **2012**, *83*, 869–873. [CrossRef]
5. Madar, J.; Roehr, C.C.; Ainsworth, S.; Ersdal, H.; Morley, C.; Rudiger, M.; Skare, C.; Szczapa, T.; Te Pas, A.; Trevisanuto, D.; et al. European resuscitation council guidelines 2021: Newborn resuscitation and support of transition of infants at birth. *Resuscitation* **2021**, *161*, 291–326. [CrossRef]
6. Klingenberg, C.; Sobotka, K.S.; Ong, T.; Allison, B.J.; Schmolzer, G.M.; Moss, T.J.; Polglase, G.R.; Dawson, J.A.; Davis, P.G.; Hooper, S.B. Effect of sustained inflation duration; resuscitation of near-term asphyxiated lambs. *Arch. Dis. Child. Fetal. Neonatal. Ed.* **2013**, *98*, F222–F227. [CrossRef]
7. Schmolzer, G.M.; O'Reilly, M.; Labossiere, J.; Lee, T.F.; Cowan, S.; Qin, S.; Bigam, D.L.; Cheung, P.Y. Cardiopulmonary resuscitation with chest compressions during sustained inflations: A new technique of neonatal resuscitation that improves recovery and survival in a neonatal porcine model. *Circulation* **2013**, *128*, 2495–2503. [CrossRef]
8. Vali, P.; Chandrasekharan, P.; Rawat, M.; Gugino, S.; Koenigsknecht, C.; Helman, J.; Mathew, B.; Berkelhamer, S.; Nair, J.; Lakshminrusimha, S. Continuous chest compressions during sustained inflations in a perinatal asphyxial cardiac arrest lamb model. *Pediatr. Crit. Care Med.* **2017**, *18*, e370–e377. [CrossRef] [PubMed]
9. Bhatt, S.; Alison, B.J.; Wallace, E.M.; Crossley, K.J.; Gill, A.W.; Kluckow, M.; te Pas, A.B.; Morley, C.J.; Polglase, G.R.; Hooper, S.B. Delaying cord clamping until ventilation onset improves cardiovascular function at birth in preterm lambs. *J. Physiol.* **2013**, *591*, 2113–2126. [CrossRef]
10. Vali, P.; Gugino, S.; Koenigsknecht, C.; Helman, J.; Chandrasekharan, P.; Rawat, M.; Lakshminrusimha, S.; Nair, J. The perinatal asphyxiated lamb model: A model for newborn resuscitation. *J. Vis. Exp.* **2018**, *138*, 57553. [CrossRef] [PubMed]
11. Aziz, K.; Lee, H.C.; Escobedo, M.B.; Hoover, A.V.; Kamath-Rayne, B.D.; Kapadia, V.S.; Magid, D.J.; Niermeyer, S.; Schmolzer, G.M.; Szyld, E.; et al. Part 5: Neonatal resuscitation: 2020 american heart association guidelines for cardiopulmonary resuscitation and emergency cardiovascular care. *Circulation* **2020**, *142*, S524–S550. [CrossRef] [PubMed]
12. Hudson, I.R.; Cavill, I.A.; Cooke, A.; Holland, B.M.; Hoy, T.G.; Trevett, D.; Turner, T.L.; Wardrop, C.A. Biotin labeling of red cells in the measurement of red cell volume in preterm infants. *Pediatr. Res.* **1990**, *28*, 199–202. [CrossRef] [PubMed]
13. Polglase, G.R.; Blank, D.A.; Barton, S.K.; Miller, S.L.; Stojanovska, V.; Kluckow, M.; Gill, A.W.; LaRosa, D.; Te Pas, A.B.; Hooper, S.B. Physiologically based cord clamping stabilises cardiac output and reduces cerebrovascular injury in asphyxiated near-term lambs. *Arch. Dis. Child. Fetal. Neonatal. Ed.* **2018**, *103*, F530–F538. [CrossRef] [PubMed]
14. Andersson, O.; Rana, N.; Ewald, U.; Malqvist, M.; Stripple, G.; Basnet, O.; Subedi, K.; Kc, A. Intact cord resuscitation versus early cord clamping in the treatment of depressed newborn infants during the first 10 min of birth (nepcord III)—A randomized clinical trial. *Matern. Health Neonatol. Perinatol.* **2019**, *5*, 15. [CrossRef]
15. Vyas, H.; Milner, A.D.; Hopkin, I.E.; Boon, A.W. Physiologic responses to prolonged and slow-rise inflation in the resuscitation of the asphyxiated newborn infant. *J. Pediatr.* **1981**, *99*, 635–639. [CrossRef]
16. Lista, G.; Boni, L.; Scopesi, F.; Mosca, F.; Trevisanuto, D.; Messner, H.; Vento, G.; Magaldi, R.; Del Vecchio, A.; Agosti, M.; et al. Sustained lung inflation at birth for preterm infants: A randomized clinical trial. *Pediatrics* **2015**, *135*, e457–e464. [CrossRef]
17. Kirpalani, H.; Ratcliffe, S.J.; Keszler, M.; Davis, P.G.; Foglia, E.E.; Te Pas, A.; Fernando, M.; Chaudhary, A.; Localio, R.; van Kaam, A.H.; et al. Effect of sustained inflations vs intermittent positive pressure ventilation on bronchopulmonary dysplasia or death among extremely preterm infants: The sail randomized clinical trial. *JAMA* **2019**, *321*, 1165–1175. [CrossRef]
18. Brouwer, E.; Te Pas, A.B.; Polglase, G.R.; McGillick, E.V.; Bohringer, S.; Crossley, K.J.; Rodgers, K.; Blank, D.; Yamaoka, S.; Gill, A.W.; et al. Effect of spontaneous breathing on umbilical venous blood flow and placental transfusion during delayed cord clamping in preterm lambs. *Arch. Dis. Child. Fetal. Neonatal. Ed.* **2020**, *105*, 26–32. [CrossRef]
19. Feihl, F.; Eckert, P.; Brimioulle, S.; Jacobs, O.; Schaller, M.D.; Melot, C.; Naeije, R. Permissive hypercapnia impairs pulmonary gas exchange in the acute respiratory distress syndrome. *Am. J. Respir. Crit. Care Med.* **2000**, *162*, 209–215. [CrossRef]
20. Polglase, G.R.; Schmolzer, G.M.; Roberts, C.T.; Blank, D.A.; Badurdeen, S.; Crossley, K.J.; Miller, S.L.; Stojanovska, V.; Galinsky, R.; Kluckow, M.; et al. Cardiopulmonary resuscitation of asystolic newborn lambs prior to umbilical cord clamping; the timing of cord clamping matters! *Front. Physiol.* **2020**, *11*, 902. [CrossRef]
21. Katheria, A.C.; Rich, W.D.; Bava, S.; Lakshminrusimha, S. Placental transfusion for asphyxiated infants. *Front Pediatr.* **2019**, *7*, 473. [CrossRef] [PubMed]
22. Linderkamp, O. Placental transfusion: Determinants and effects. *Clin. Perinatol.* **1982**, *9*, 559–592. [CrossRef]
23. Katheria, A.C.; Lakshminrusimha, S.; Rabe, H.; McAdams, R.; Mercer, J.S. Placental transfusion: A review. *J. Perinatol.* **2017**, *37*, 105–111. [CrossRef] [PubMed]
24. Creasy, R.K.; Drost, M.; Green, M.V.; Morris, J.A. Effect of ventilation on transfer of blood from placenta to neonate. *Am. J. Physiol.* **1972**, *222*, 186–188. [CrossRef]

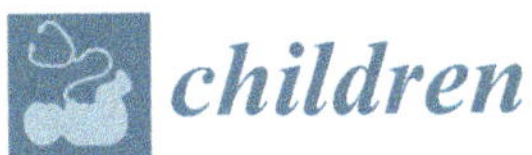

Article

The Assisted Breathing before Cord Clamping (ABC) Study Protocol

Michael P. Meyer [1,2,*] and Elizabeth Nevill [1]

1   Neonatal Unit, KidzFirst, Middlemore Hospital, Auckland 2025, New Zealand; elizabeth.nevill@cmdhb.org.nz
2   Department of Paediatrics, University of Auckland, Auckland 2025, New Zealand
*   Correspondence: michael.meyer@middlemore.co.nz

Abstract: Major physiologic changes occur during the transition after birth. For preterm infants, current understanding favours allowing the initial changes to occur prior to cord clamping. Amongst other improved outcomes, systematic reviews have indicated a significant reduction in neonatal blood transfusions following delayed cord clamping. This may be due to a placental transfusion, facilitated by the onset of respiration. If breathing is compromised, placental transfusion may be reduced, resulting in a greater red cell transfusion rate. We designed a randomised trial to investigate whether assisting respiration in this high-risk group of babies would decrease blood transfusion and improve outcomes. The Assisted Breathing before Cord Clamping (ABC) study is a single-centre randomised controlled trial. Preterm infants < 31 weeks that have not established regular breathing before 15 s are randomised to a standard or intervention group. The intervention is intermittent positive pressure ventilation via T piece for 30 s, whilst standard management consists of 30 s of positioning and gentle stimulation. The cord is clamped at 50 s in both groups. The primary outcome is the proportion of infants in each group receiving blood transfusion during the neonatal admission. Secondary outcomes include requirement for resuscitation, the assessment of circulatory status and neonatal outcomes.

Keywords: preterm; delayed cord clamping; resuscitation; clinical trial; protocol; red blood cell transfusion; preterm cardiovascular transition

Citation: Meyer, M.P.; Nevill, E. The Assisted Breathing before Cord Clamping (ABC) Study Protocol. *Children* **2021**, *8*, 336. https://doi.org/10.3390/children8050336

Academic Editor: Simone Pratesi

Received: 31 March 2021
Accepted: 21 April 2021
Published: 26 April 2021

1. Introduction

Major physiologic changes occur during the transition immediately after birth. These include lung aeration and expansion, which is associated with a marked and rapid reduction in pulmonary vascular resistance and increased pulmonary blood flow [1]. This changes the direction of the ductal shunt so that it is primarily left to right, and the systemic blood flow is largely derived from the increased left ventricular output. The in utero vascular resistance is low because of the placental bed. Cord clamping has the potential to change this vascular resistance, particularly if the lungs have not been expanded [2,3]. Preterm infants, who may not rapidly establish adequate lung aeration before cord clamping, are at a high risk of perturbations to this normal process especially if the cord is clamped early. Indeed, clamping the preterm cord after a delay of at least 30 s has been shown in a number of systematic reviews to improve survival, although this finding was recently noted to be of borderline significance [4–6]. As noted above, however, the critical factor in the timing of the cord clamping may be related to the onset of respiration rather than the time elapsed. Whilst this was suggested years ago [7,8], there has been a recent resurgence of studies examining "physiologic" cord clamping once breathing is fully established [9,10]. To date, most of these studies are small feasibility studies, although larger clinical studies are underway or have been proposed [11]. If the cord is not clamped immediately (or "early") and clamping is "deferred" or "delayed" (DCC) for a period of time (e.g., 30 to 60 s), many infants, including those that are very preterm, will be breathing before clamping. In a recent study of infants < 32 weeks, this amounted to approximately 70% at 30 s and 90% by 60 s [12,13]. On the other hand, if preterm infants are not breathing before clamping, they may be deemed to be in need of resuscitation, hence the term "neonatal resuscitation with an intact cord" [1].

The finding of some importance and consistency in meta-analysis in relation to DCC in preterm infants is a reduction in neonatal blood transfusion. The overall relative risk for DCC compared to early clamping was 0.81 (0.74–0.87) with moderate heterogeneity (61%). For infants < 28 weeks, the risk was 0.91 (0.85–0.97) with 39% heterogeneity [4]. The mean haematocrit increase in the DCC group was 2.7%. The largest study included in the meta-analysis contributed to over 50% of the cases and showed a significant reduction of 10% in the proportion of infants transfused [14]. The other relatively large study was the UK Cord Trial [15], where infants < 32 weeks were randomised to 2 min or more DCC compared to clamping before 20 s. Neonatal outcomes were assessed in 266 infants with a similar reduction in the proportion of transfused infants from 54 to 47%, although this difference was not significant. The number of infants transfused for early hypotension in this study was, however, significantly decreased from 6/132 to 0/134 ($p = 0. 014$).

Although the reasons for neonatal transfusion are multifactorial, there is evidence of a transfer of blood from the placenta (a placental transfusion) to the infant in cases where DCC occurs, and this may be one mechanism for the observed reduction in neonatal transfusions. Although a few studies have directly measured the infant's blood volume, most of the evidence for placental transfusion is indirect [16,17]. There is an increase in haematocrit in many randomised trials (where the control group did not have DCC), an increase in body weight demonstrated by continuous weighing after birth with the cord intact and a corresponding decrease in placental weight compared to cases where no DCC occurred [4,16,18]. In addition, many earlier studies measured the residual placental blood volume (RPV) by allowing blood from the placenta to drain under gravity into a graduated measuring cylinder after delivery [19], DCC was associated with a reduction in the RPV. Important factors determining the RPV, i.e., the inferred amount of placental transfusion, were whether breathing occurred during DCC and the length of time after birth before the cord was clamped. In term infants, it appeared that the initial cry was enough to facilitate placental transfusion, as the majority of the decrease in RPV occurred quickly, even if breathing was not sustained. In preterm infants, however, this placental transfusion appeared to take longer, possibly associated with a reduced respiratory effort [19,20]. In addition, the length of DCC may be curtailed because of the desire of attending staff to start early resuscitation, particularly if early respiration is not vigorous. The effect of this shorter duration of DCC combined with irregular respiration on placental transfusion is not clear. Such infants may have been excluded from randomised trials (approximately 20% in the two largest studies) [14,15]. In an observational study of infants < 30 weeks carried out at our hospital, of 46 infants undergoing DCC (40 s or more), 34 established regular breathing during the procedure, whilst 12 (26%) did not. Sixty percent of infants that received DCC and did not breathe received an RBC transfusion compared to 32% in the group that breathed regularly. The median day 1 haemoglobin was significantly higher in this latter group ($p = 0.003$). These differences suggest a larger placental transfusion in the group that breathed during DCC even though the length of DCC was similar [21]. This led us to question whether providing respiratory support to preterm infants who did not establish regular breathing during DCC (but were not otherwise compromised) would allow a greater placental transfusion to take place and subsequently reduce neonatal blood transfusion requirements. We estimated that the assessment and randomisation could be completed within 20 s of birth and planned a further 30 s of DCC, with 1:1 randomisation to either receive respiratory support or no respiratory support during the last 30 s. All study infants would receive a total of 50 s DCC. In PICOT format, this was as follows:

P preterm infants < 31 weeks undergoing DCC who did not establish regular respiration by 15 s were randomised to the

I intervention of the T piece intermittent positive pressure ventilation (IPPV) with 30% oxygen compared to the

C control group who received standard care during DCC without IPPV.

O outcome assessment was blood transfusion.

T time during the neonatal admission.

We anticipated several problems with the study implementation:

Ergonomics: Birth, and particularly very preterm birth, is a stressful time with space and equipment limitations. Other investigators have used purpose-built resuscitation trolleys, radiant warmers or other surfaces for infant assessment and management [12,22,23]. However, as described in the "Methods", we used heated towels on the mother's thighs or placed the infant at the foot of the bed for vaginal births. We had one skilled operator in charge of the infant who stood next to the surgeon, and in our preliminary trials, this pragmatic approach was satisfactory.

Monitoring: Ideally, heart rate and pulse oximetry and temperature should be continuously monitored during this short transition. A recent study found dry electrodes to be the quickest tool for monitoring heart rate (median 13 s) followed by ECG (42 s) and pulse oximetry (105 s). The dry gel electrodes for preterm infants are not yet commercially available and the other methods are too slow for this short period [9,24]. Similarly, with only one neonatal attendee, we could not routinely auscultate or palpate the heart rate. This meant we had to rely on the observation of breathing, activity, tone and colour for monitoring.

Sterility: Apart from the neonatal attendee who wore sterile theatre attire, the only contact with the sterile field was the sterile plastic wrap, respiratory circuit and T-piece. A local supplier was able to gas sterilise these components for caesarean deliveries.

Randomisation and time: The decision to randomise was undertaken at 15 s and intervention was started by 20 s (this is described in detail below). In simulation testing, we could achieve this with opaque sealed numbered envelopes if we used a colour coded card in the envelope. One of the reasons we did not want to prolong the total DCC time beyond 50 s was because of the safety of the mother and difficulties of safely monitoring potentially compromised infants.

Temperature: We applied the sterile thermal wrap immediately after delivery but no other form of heating until the infant was placed under the radiant warmer after cord clamping.

Efficacy of respiratory support: Studies have shown T-piece IPPV may be ineffective in delivering adequate tidal volumes in preterm infants, possibly because of an air leak or a closed glottis [25,26]. To help assess respiration, we inserted a colorimetric carbon dioxide detector into the circuit.

Outcome/sample size: We calculated a sample size as described in the Methods section. This was based on our previous observational study. Our neonatal blood transfusion guidelines are restrictive and as the day-to-day attending staff were blinded as to whether the infant received the intervention or not, randomisation was expected to reduce bias in deciding whether blood transfusion was indicated.

Recruitment: We surmised that either antenatal or deferred consent were required to achieve a realistic study population. Previous studies in our hospital indicated that restricting the study to those with antenatal consent was likely to mean that >50% of potential cases were ineligible.

2. ABC Study Protocol

The Assisted Breathing before Cord Clamping study (The ABC Study) (http://www.anzctr.org.au/ACTRN12615001026516.aspx, accessed on 28 January 2020) protocol is described below in more detail. The study design was a single centre randomised controlled trial at a New Zealand centre that had first implemented DCC in 2010. On average 70 < 31 weeks infants are admitted per year, and it was estimated that 50% of infants undergoing DCC would not be breathing regularly by 15 s [13].

2.1. Eligibility

Inclusion criteria: Infants < 31 weeks gestation delivered vaginally or by caesarean section and undergoing DCC are eligible once their breathing has been assessed at 15 s of age and the infant is deemed not to have regular rhythmic breathing (chest wall movement).

2.2. Exclusion Criteria

- Obstetric reasons: Declined antenatal consent, severe antenatal intrauterine growth restriction (estimated foetal weight < 10th customised centile), twin-to-twin transfusion syndrome, maternal compromise, abruption, en caul, short cord, known severe congenital abnormality.
- Infant reasons: Established regular breathing by 15 s, compromised and in need of immediate resuscitation (apnoeic, flaccid, pale).

2.3. Interventions

Infants that receive DCC are eligible for randomisation at 15 s of age if breathing (chest wall movement) appears irregular or absent, but the infant is not otherwise compromised (see below). A control group receiving standard treatment will be compared to an intervention arm. Standard treatment consists of the infant being placed supine with the head in a neutral breathing position, placed in a thermal wrap whilst receiving gentle stimulation (face dried, touching or rubbing the torso or back) and completing 50 s DCC. Infants randomised to the intervention arm will receive breathing support in the form of intermittent positive pressure ventilation (IPPV) and continuous positive airway pressure (CPAP) delivered by appropriate mask and T-Piece in addition to standard treatment as described above (Figure 1).

The designated resuscitation team leader (RTL) will collect a sealed, numbered, stratified randomisation envelope for eligible infants < 31 weeks and discuss the study with the midwife and obstetric team antenatally or before delivery.

2.4. Equipment

For vaginal deliveries, the T-piece pressure-controlled device (Neopuff, Fisher & Paykel, Auckland, New Zealand) attached to the heat table (Giraffe Warmer, GE Healthcare, Auckland, New Zealand) will be used; the heat table will be lowered to minimum height, next to that of the delivery bed, to allow the circuit and T-piece to reach the foot of the maternal bed. A colorimetric device (Pedicap, Covidien^{TM}, Mansfield, MA, USA) will be inserted into the T-piece circuit. A sterile thermal body wrap will be used (Fisher & Paykel, Auckland, New Zealand). Time keeping will be done using the Apgar score timer.

Caesarean section deliveries require sterile consumables, i.e., sterile mask and T-piece circuit, sterile thermal wrap and a colorimetric device. The T-piece and gas blender (without humidity) are attached to a mobile pendant located in the obstetric theatre and checked. The RTL will adhere to surgical protocols.

The T-piece settings include gas flow 10 L/min, set pressure 20/5 cm water and FiO_2 0.3. The colorimetric device will be placed between the T-piece and mask.

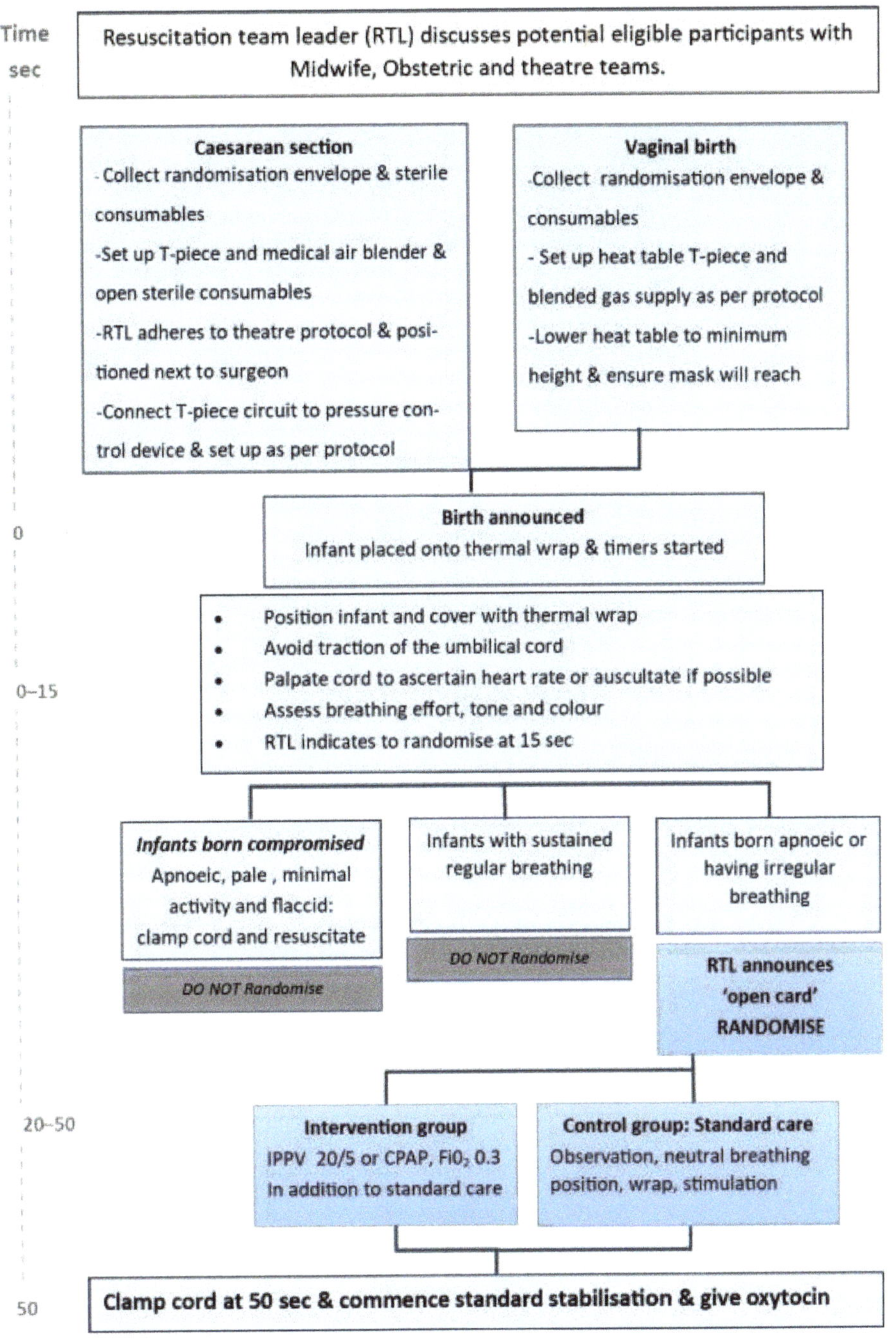

Figure 1. ABC Study flow diagram.

2.5. Procedure

Time keeping: Timers will be started when "baby out" is announced. The research assistant will call out "15 s" and the RTL will respond by announcing "open/randomise" or indicate not to open the randomisation card once the breathing has been assessed. The research assistant will announce when 50 s has elapsed to clamp the cord.

Randomisation will take place after applying thermal wrap, placing infant supine in a neutral position (see above) and assessing breathing as follows:

- Apnoeic infants or those that do not have sustained respiratory effort but no pallor and appear well perfused with reasonable tone are eligible.
- Infants born compromised (apneic, pale, flaccid) and deemed in need of immediate resuscitation are not eligible and have the cord clamped and standard resuscitation commenced [27].

Infants who appear vigorous, with sustained breathing (chest wall movement) at 15 s of age are not eligible for randomisation and neither are infants who initially establish respiration and then became apnoeic after 15 s.

Standard treatment is indicated by a white laminated card whilst the intervention arm is indicated by a blue laminated card (intervention as previously described). During the 50 s DCC, the procedure may be terminated for safety concerns (abruption, clinical deterioration of the mother or infant). After the cord is cut, the infant is placed into a sterile cot (caesarean section) and transferred to a heat table; after vaginal births, the infant will be placed directly onto the heat table. The attending RTL performs the procedure for multiples and a second attendant continues cares after the completion of cord clamping. Oxytocin is to be given after the completion of 50 s DCC for all deliveries as per standard obstetric practice. Standard delivery room management includes humidified Hudson bubble CPAP (6–8 cm; Fisher & Paykel, Auckland, New Zealand) skin servo temperature control, heart rate and saturation monitoring.

2.6. Outcome Measures

The primary outcome is red blood cell transfusion rates during the neonatal admission. The proportion of infants transfused as well as the number of transfusions and volume of blood transfused will be compared, with the primary comparison being the proportion transfused in either group. The study centre transfusion guideline will remain unchanged during the planned study period (Table A1 in Appendix A). Infants who receive a transfusion at a surgical centre will be recorded separately to avoid the problem of differing blood transfusion guidelines.

2.7. Secondary Outcomes

- Apgar scores and delivery room resuscitation including the requirement for endotracheal intubation.
- Core axillary temperature (digital electronic thermometer) at 5 min of age and on admission to NICU.
- Respiratory support including surfactant, length and type of support.
- Transitional circulation assessed based on blood pressure recorded from arterial lines where possible or peripheral recordings if no arterial lines, acid base, lactate, echocardiogram performed within first 6–12 h if possible, inotropes received (first 48 h) and patent ductus arteriosus treatment rates during neonatal admission.
- Phototherapy received (requirement based on local guidelines) haemoglobin levels on days 1 at 24 h of age and days 2, 3 and 7 (from capillary or venous FBC as preference or capillary gas).
- Neonatal outcomes as defined by local neonatal network coding criteria [28]. These include: chronic lung disease (CLD) defined as respiratory support or oxygen received at 36 weeks corrected gestational age, discharge home with oxygen, intraventricular haemorrhage (IVH) rates (grades III and IV and any grade reported) within first 24 h if possible, day 5 and day 28 cranial ultrasound, necrotising enterocolitis (NEC) defined

by modified Bells stage 2 or higher, retinopathy of prematurity (ROP) highest stage recorded and requiring laser therapy, early onset sepsis (EOS) < 48 h of age and late onset sepsis (LOS) defined by positive blood culture or cerebrospinal fluid after 48 h, death during neonatal admission and length of hospital stay in days [28].

- Neurodevelopmental outcome at 2 years of age (for infants $\leq$ 29 week gestation).

2.8. Sample Size

Data from an observational study indicated that 60% of infants that received DCC and did not breathe received a blood transfusion. This compared to 30% transfused in the group that breathed during DCC. Aiming for a similar 50% relative reduction in the proportion transfused would require 100 infants whose primary outcome could be assessed. To allow for cases where outcome assessment may not be possible (deaths, surgical transfer), 120 infants are to be randomised (60 per group). (A total of 100 would give the study 85% power at a two-sided significance level of 0.05). For a secondary composite outcome of death, CLD or severe IVH, the sample size would allow a 36% difference in outcome to be detected (80% power, significance 0.05), assuming the percentage of infants with a composite endpoint will be 58% (based on historic data).

2.9. Intervention Assignment

Sequence generation: One-to-one allocation to study groups based on computer generated randomisation sequences with random block sizes. Groups will be stratified into $\leq$26, >26 and <28 weeks and $\geq$28 to <31 weeks gestation.

2.10. Concealment Mechanism

Randomisation will occur via sequentially numbered brown opaque sealed envelopes containing laminated colour cards to reveal the intervention. The colour code cannot be determined without opening the envelope. Multiples will be randomised as individual participants.

2.11. Implementation

The envelope will only be opened once the resuscitation team leader instructs the research assistant to do so. The infants study number will be documented on the birth record and delivery data collection sheet.

2.12. Masking

The laminated coloured card and completed randomisation data sheet will be placed in a secure box located in a locked office (only accessible to the research nurse collecting and entering the blinded data into a secure data base). Outcome assessment will be carried out by members of the study team without knowledge of the intervention group.

2.13. Data Management

Standardised data collection forms are entered into Research Electronic Data Capture (REDCap, Vanderbilt University Medical Centre, Institute for Clinical and Translational Research, hosted by University of Auckland, Auckland, New Zealand) by an administrator [29].

A data safety monitoring committee (DSMC) was established.

2.14. Statistics

Initial chi-square tests for categorical data. Numeric data are to be analysed with Mann–Whitney non-parametric statistics or t test if normally distributed. Secondary analysis is planned using logistic regression (IBM SPSS Statistics 26, IBM Corporation 2020, New York, NY, USA). Two-sided probability (*p* value) < 0.05 will be used to indicate statistical significance.

2.15. Ethics

Written informed consent will be obtained before labour where possible. In cases where active labour is in progress; and consent before birth is not possible, approval was obtained from the Northern A Health and Disability Ethics Committee, New Zealand (15/NTA/146AM01) as well as the following local groups to allow randomisation at birth, and obtain postnatal consent for the collection of outcome data: Māori Health Ethics committee, Patient Whanau Centred Care Consumer Council, Maternity consumer group, organisational legal opinion, parental input from Neonatal Unit parents of preterm infants as well as Neonatal, Midwifery, Obstetric and Anaesthetic department stakeholders. In cases where antenatal consent could not be obtained and parents decline consent, the initial data capture sheet will be discarded, and no further data collected.

Author Contributions: Conceptualisation, M.P.M. and E.N.; methodology, M.P.M. and E.N.; writing—original draft preparation, M.P.M. and E.N.; writing—review and editing, M.P.M. and E.N.; visualisation, E.N.; supervision, M.P.M.; project administration, M.P.M. and E.N.; funding acquisition, E.N. All authors have read and agreed to the published version of the manuscript.

Funding: This research was funded by Middlemore Hospital Research Fund, Tupu Grant and the APC was funded by Neonatal Research Fund, Middlemore Hospital.

Institutional Review Board Statement: The study was conducted according to the guidelines of the Declaration of Helsinki and approved by the National Ethics Committee of New Zealand (protocol code 15/NTA/146).

Informed Consent Statement: Informed consent was obtained from all subjects involved in the study.

Conflicts of Interest: The authors declare no conflict of interest. The funders had no role in the design of the study; in the collection, analyses, or interpretation of data; in the writing of the manuscript, or in the decision to publish the results.

Appendix A

Table A1. Hospital blood transfusion guideline.

Haemoglobin (Hb) (Haematocrit)	Consider Transfusion
Hb < 70 g/L (Haematocrit $\leq$ 20%)	Symptomatic anaemia: any of the following without obvious cause: • Significant apnoea and bradycardia while receiving caffeine (>9 episodes in 12 h or 2 episodes in 24 h requiring bag mask ventilation). • Heart rate > 170 beats per minute or respiration rate > 70 breaths per minute persists for 24 h. • Poor weight gain (< 10g/day over 7 days). • Increasing ductal shunt and cardiac decompensation. Any positive pressure support. Asymptomatic with reticulocytes < 100,000 $\times$ 10^9/L.
Hb 70–80 g/L (Haematocrit 21–25%)	Symptomatic anaemia as above. CPAP with FiO_2 0.25–0.4. Undergoing surgery.
Hb 81–100 g/L (Haematocrit $\leq$ 25–30%)	CPAP with FiO_2 > 0.4. Mechanical ventilation with MAP $\geq$ 7–10 cm H_2O.
Hb 101–110 g/L (Haematocrit $\leq$ 21–25%)	Critically unwell with one or more of the following: • CPAP and FiO_2 > 0.4. • Ventilation MAP > 10 cm H_2O. • Acute bleeding.

References

1. Dawes, G.S.; Mott, J.C.; Widdicombe, J.G.; Wyatt, D.G. Changes in the lungs of the newborn lamb. *J. Physiol.* **1953**, *121*, 141–162. [CrossRef] [PubMed]
2. Bhatt, S.; Alison, B.J.; Wallace, E.M.; Crossley, K.J.; Gill, A.W.; Kluckow, M.; Te Pas, A.B.; Morley, C.J.; Polglase, G.R.; Hooper, S.B. Delaying cord clamping until ventilation onset improves cardiovascular function at birth in preterm lambs. *J. Physiol.* **2013**, *591*, 2113–2126. [CrossRef]
3. Hooper, S.B.; Polglase, G.R.; Pas, A.B.T. A physiological approach to the timing of umbilical cord clamping at birth. *Arch. Dis. Child. Fetal Neonatal Ed.* **2015**, *100*, F355–F360. [CrossRef]
4. Fogarty, M.; Osborn, D.A.; Askie, L.; Seidler, A.L.; Hunter, K.; Lui, K.; Simes, J.; Tarnow-Mordi, W. Delayed vs early umbilical cord clamping for preterm infants: A systematic review and meta-analysis. *Am. J. Obstet. Gynecol.* **2018**, *218*, 1–18. [CrossRef]
5. Rabe, H.; Gyte, G.M.; Díaz-Rossello, J.L.; Duley, L. Effect of timing of umbilical cord clamping and other strategies to influence placental transfusion at preterm birth on maternal and infant outcomes. *Cochrane Database Syst. Rev.* **2019**, *2019*, CD003248. [CrossRef] [PubMed]
6. Seidler, A.L.; Gyte, G.M.; Rabe, H.; Díaz-Rossello, J.L.; Duley, L.; Aziz, K.; Costa-Nobre, D.T.; Davis, P.G.; Schmölzer, G.M.; Ovelman, C.; et al. Umbilical Cord Management for Newborns <34 Weeks' Gestation: A Meta-analysis. *Pediatrics* **2021**, *147*, e20200576. [CrossRef]
7. Brown, R.J.K. Respiratory Difficulties at Birth. *BMJ* **1959**, *1*, 404–408. [CrossRef] [PubMed]
8. Darwin, E. Zoonomia; Or, The Laws of Organic Life: In Four Volumes. *J. Johns. St. Paul's Church Yard* **1801**, *2*, 302.
9. Blank, D.A.; Badurdeen, S.; Kamlin, C.O.F.; Jacobs, S.E.; Thio, M.; Dawson, J.A.; Kane, S.C.; Dennis, A.T.; Polglase, G.R.; Hooper, S.B.; et al. Baby-directed umbilical cord clamping: A feasibility study. *Resuscitation* **2018**, *131*, 1–7. [CrossRef]
10. Knol, R.; Brouwer, E.; Akker, T.V.D.; DeKoninck, P.; van Geloven, N.; Polglase, G.R.; Lopriore, E.; Herkert, E.; Reiss, I.K.; Hooper, S.B.; et al. Physiological-based cord clamping in very preterm infants—Randomised controlled trial on effectiveness of stabilisation. *Resuscitation* **2020**, *147*, 26–33. [CrossRef]
11. Katheria, A.C. Neonatal Resuscitation with an Intact Cord: Current and Ongoing Trials. *Children* **2019**, *6*, 60. [CrossRef]
12. Katheria, A.; Poeltler, D.; Durham, J.; Steen, J.; Rich, W.; Arnell, K.; Maldonado, M.; Cousins, L.; Finer, N. Neonatal Resuscitation with an Intact Cord: A Randomized Clinical Trial. *J. Pediatr.* **2016**, *178*, 75–80.e3. [CrossRef] [PubMed]
13. Katheria, A.C.; Lakshminrusimha, S.; Rabe, H.; McAdams, R.; Mercer, J.S. Placental transfusion: A review. *J. Perinatol.* **2017**, *37*, 105–111. [CrossRef] [PubMed]
14. Tarnow-Mordi, W.; Morris, J.; Kirby, A.; Robledo, K.; Askie, L.; Brown, R.; Evans, N.; Finlayson, S.; Fogarty, M.; Gebski, V.; et al. Delayed versus Immediate Cord Clamping in Preterm Infants. *N. Engl. J. Med.* **2017**, *377*, 2445–2455. [CrossRef] [PubMed]
15. Duley, L.; Dorling, J.; Pushpa-Rajah, A.; Oddie, S.J.; Yoxall, C.W.; Schoonakker, B.; Bradshaw, L.; Mitchell, E.J.; Fawke, J.A. Randomised trial of cord clamping and initial stabilisation at very preterm birth. *Arch. Dis. Child. Fetal Neonatal Ed.* **2017**, *103*, F6–F14. [CrossRef] [PubMed]
16. Moss, A.J.; Monset-Couchard, M. Placental transfusion: Early versus late clamping of the umbilical cord. *Pediatrics* **1967**, *40*, 109–126. [PubMed]
17. Aladangady, N.; McHugh, S.; Aitchison, T.C.; Wardrop, C.A.J.; Holland, B.M. Infants' Blood Volume in a Controlled Trial of Placental Transfusion at Preterm Delivery. *Pediatrics* **2006**, *117*, 93–98. [CrossRef] [PubMed]
18. Farrar, D.; Airey, R.; Law, G.R.; Tuffnell, D.; Cattle, B.; Duley, L. Measuring placental transfusion for term births: Weighing babies with cord intact. *BJOG* **2010**, *118*, 70–75. [CrossRef]
19. Redmond, A.; Isana, S.; Ingall, D. Relation of onset of respiration to placental transfusion. *Obstet. Gynecol. Surv.* **1965**, *20*, 781–783. [CrossRef]
20. Kjeldsen, J.; Pedersen, J. Relation of residual placental blood-volume to onset of respiration and the respiratory-distress syndrome in infants of diabetic and non-diabetic mothers. *Lancet* **1967**, *289*, 180–184. [CrossRef]
21. Nevill, E.; Meyer, M.P. Effect of delayed cord clamping (DCC) on breathing and transition at birth in very preterm infants. *Early Hum. Dev.* **2015**, *91*, 407–411. [CrossRef]
22. Thomas, M.R.; Yoxall, C.W.; Weeks, A.D.; Duley, L. Providing newborn resuscitation at the mother's bedside: Assessing the safety, usability and acceptability of a mobile trolley. *BMC Pediatr.* **2014**, *14*, 135. [CrossRef]
23. Brouwer, E.; Knol, R.; Vernooij, A.S.N.; Akker, T.V.D.; Vlasman, P.E.; Klumper, F.J.C.M.; Dekoninck, P.; Polglase, G.R.; Hooper, S.B.; Pas, A.B.T. Physiological-based cord clamping in preterm infants using a new purpose-built resuscitation table: A feasibility study. *Arch. Dis. Child. Fetal Neonatal Ed.* **2018**, *104*, F396–F402. [CrossRef] [PubMed]
24. Bush, J.B.; Cooley, V.; Perlman, J.; Chang, C. NeoBeat offers rapid newborn heart rate assessment. *Arch. Dis. Child. Fetal Neonatal Ed.* **2021**. [CrossRef]
25. Harding, R.; Hooper, S.B. Regulation of lung expansion and lung growth before birth. *J. Appl. Physiol.* **1996**, *81*, 209–224. [CrossRef] [PubMed]
26. van Vonderen, J.J.; Hooper, S.B.; Hummler, H.D.; Lopriore, E.; Pas, A.B.T. Effects of a Sustained Inflation in Preterm Infants at Birth. *J. Pediatr.* **2014**, *165*, 903–908.e1. [CrossRef]
27. Perlman, J.M.; Wyllie, J.; Kattwinkel, J.; Wyckoff, M.H.; Aziz, K.; Guinsburg, R.; Kim, H.-S.; Liley, H.G.; Mildenhall, L.; Simon, W.M.; et al. Part 7: Neonatal resuscitation: 2015 international consensus on cardiopulmonary resuscitation and emergency cardiovascular care science with treatment recommendations. *Circulation* **2015**, *132*, S204–S241. [CrossRef]

28. Australian and New Zealand Neonatal Network; Chow, S.S.; Creighton, P.; Kander, V.; Haslam, R.; Lui, K. Report of the Australian and New Zealand Neonatal Network, 2016. *J. Paediatr. Child Health* **2018**. [CrossRef]
29. Harris, P.A.; Taylor, R.; Thielke, R.; Payne, J.; Gonzalez, N.; Conde, J.G. Research electronic data capture (REDCap)—A metadata-driven methodology and workflow process for providing translational research informatics support. *J. Biomed. Inform.* **2009**, *42*, 377–381. [CrossRef]

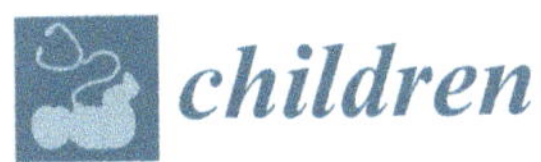

Article

The BabySaver: Design of a New Device for Neonatal Resuscitation at Birth with Intact Placental Circulation

James Ditai [1,2,3,*], Aisling Barry [4], Kathy Burgoine [5], Anthony K. Mbonye [6], Julius N. Wandabwa [3], Peter Watt [7] and Andrew D. Weeks [2]

1   Sanyu Africa Research Institute, Mbale Regional Referral Hospital, Pallisa Road, Mbale P.O. Box 2190, Uganda
2   Sanyu Research Unit, Department of Women's and Children's Health, University of Liverpool, Liverpool Women's Hospital, Crown Street, Liverpool L8 7SS, UK; aweeks@liv.ac.uk
3   Faculty of Health Sciences, Busitema University, Pallisa Road, Mbale P.O. Box 2190, Uganda; gjwandabwa@yahoo.com
4   The Department of Medical Engineering and Physics, Kings College London, London SE5 9RS, UK; aislingfbarry@gmail.com
5   Neonatal Unit, Mbale Regional Referral Hospital, Pallisa Road, Mbale P.O. Box 2190, Uganda; Kathy.burgoine@liv.ac.uk
6   School of Public Health, Makerere University College of Health Sciences, Kampala P.O. Box 7072, Uganda; akmbonye@yahoo.com
7   Department of Medical Physics and Clinical Engineering, University of Liverpool, Liverpool L7 8XP, UK; rjpwatt@gmail.com
*   Correspondence: j.ditai@safri.ac.ug; Tel.: +256-702-620-194

Citation: Ditai, J.; Barry, A.; Burgoine, K.; Mbonye, A.K.; Wandabwa, J.N.; Watt, P.; Weeks, A.D. The BabySaver: Design of a New Device for Neonatal Resuscitation at Birth with Intact Placental Circulation. *Children* 2021, 8, 526. https://doi.org/10.3390/children8060526

Academic Editors: Simone Pratesi, David Hutchon and Anup Katheria

Received: 29 May 2021
Accepted: 17 June 2021
Published: 21 June 2021

Publisher's Note: MDPI stays neutral with regard to jurisdictional claims in published maps and institutional affiliations.

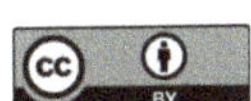

Abstract: The initial bedside care of premature babies with an intact cord has been shown to reduce mortality; there is evidence that resuscitation of term babies with an intact cord may also improve outcomes. This process has been facilitated by the development of bedside resuscitation surfaces. These new devices are unaffordable, however, in most of sub-Saharan Africa, where 42% of the world's 2.4 million annual newborn deaths occur. This paper describes the rationale and design of BabySaver, an innovative low-cost mobile resuscitation unit, which was developed iteratively over five years in a collaboration between the Sanyu Africa Research Institute (SAfRI) in Uganda and the University of Liverpool in the UK. The final BabySaver design comprises two compartments; a tray to provide a firm resuscitation surface, and a base to store resuscitation equipment. The design was formed while considering contextual factors, using the views of individual women from the community served by the local hospitals, medical staff, and skilled birth attendants in both Uganda and the UK.

Keywords: intact cord; resuscitation; placental circulation; design; BabySaver

1. Introduction

Sub-Saharan Africa is reported to have 1 million newborn deaths annually, accounting for 42% of the world's total newborn deaths [1–3]. The need for any form of resuscitation at birth is 10% globally [4] but rates are higher in sub-Saharan African countries with reported rates of 24–32% [5–7]. Most babies needing resuscitation require only simple stimulation (drying and rubbing), which can be performed at the mother's side without transferring the baby to another resuscitation surface; 3–6% of all babies (approximately 6 million/year) require further (basic) neonatal resuscitation, comprising stimulation plus bag and mask ventilation; very few need advanced resuscitation (chest compression, endotracheal intubation, and medication) [4]. It is estimated that the provision of universal access to basic resuscitation of newborns could save 904,000 newborn lives annually, with additional reductions in chronic neurological abnormalities [8]. Historically, however, the focus has been on staff training and the provision of resuscitation areas away from the mother.

Providing neonatal resuscitation at the mother's bedside with an intact umbilical cord is potentially a high benefit practice with major global benefits; it enables physiological benefits for the baby, keeps the midwife with the mother in the vital few minutes after birth, and allows the mother to stay with her newborn, preventing any suspicion of malpractice [9–11].

In the United Kingdom, Hutchon and colleagues explored ways of achieving resuscitation with an intact cord. This resulted in the development of a small mobile bedside resuscitation trolley, later commercialised as the LifeStart trolley (Inspiration Healthcare, Crawley, UK) [12–15]. This was followed in the Netherlands by Concord: a purpose-built resuscitation table for physiological-based cord clamping in preterms [16–19]. Other devices developed to date include the NOOMA cart in the USA and the INSPiRE trolley in Canada [20]. However, these innovations are not possible in low-resource settings as they require expensive equipment, a hospital base, and mains electricity.

The BabySaver is a simple mobile vacuum-moulded, oval plastic assembly resuscitation unit developed by a team of designers at the Royal Liverpool University Hospital, researchers at SAfRI, and clinicians at Liverpool Women's Hospital (LWH) and Mbale Regional Referral Hospital. It is the first medical device designed to promote neonatal resuscitation with an intact cord in low-resource settings. The final device prototype has since undergone phase I and II clinical testing studies in Uganda, reported elsewhere.

This paper discusses the rationale and design of a medical device, including the nature and effect of contextual factors on its final design.

The Rationale for the BabySaver Newborn Resuscitation Device

The primary objective for developing the BabySaver device was to reduce intrapartum-related deaths in low-resource delivery environments. We aimed to develop a device that:

- provides a stable, flat but firm surface for the baby [10] and enables the skilled birth attendant to resuscitate during the first "golden minute" after birth [21]
- facilitates resuscitation of depressed neonates at birth whilst keeping the umbilical cord intact [9–11]
- allows resuscitation of the babies by the mother's side [9–11]
- prevents separation of the skilled birth attendant and mother, so that the care of the mother is not interrupted
- allows the mother to remain with the baby during its initial support, instead of removing it from her sight during these vital moments
- facilitates newborn resuscitation when only one skilled birth attendant is present.

The BabySaver newborn resuscitation device was designed from simple plastics to maximise sustainability in Uganda's public health facilities and replicability in low-resource settings across the world.

2. Materials and Methods

2.1. Team

The design and development of the BabySaver device were coordinated by a small team of academics working within the Sanyu Research Unit, the Royal Liverpool University Hospital Department of Physics and Engineering, in collaboration with SAfRI. SAfRI is a not-for-profit non-government organisation, based at Mbale Regional Referral Hospital in Eastern Uganda; it and the Sanyu Research Unit in Liverpool were set up to research low-cost innovations and improve the care of mothers and their newborns. The team includes those who were responsible for the development of a high-end bedside resuscitation trolley for the US and European market, sold as the "Lifestart" trolley [15].

2.2. Design Process

The BabySaver underwent systematic design using the framework of engineering design [22]. The design took place in four main phases: (1) plan and clarify the task, (2) the conceptual design, (3) embodiment design, and (4) detailed design. Figure 1 shows a summary of the design process specific to the BabySaver based on this framework [22].

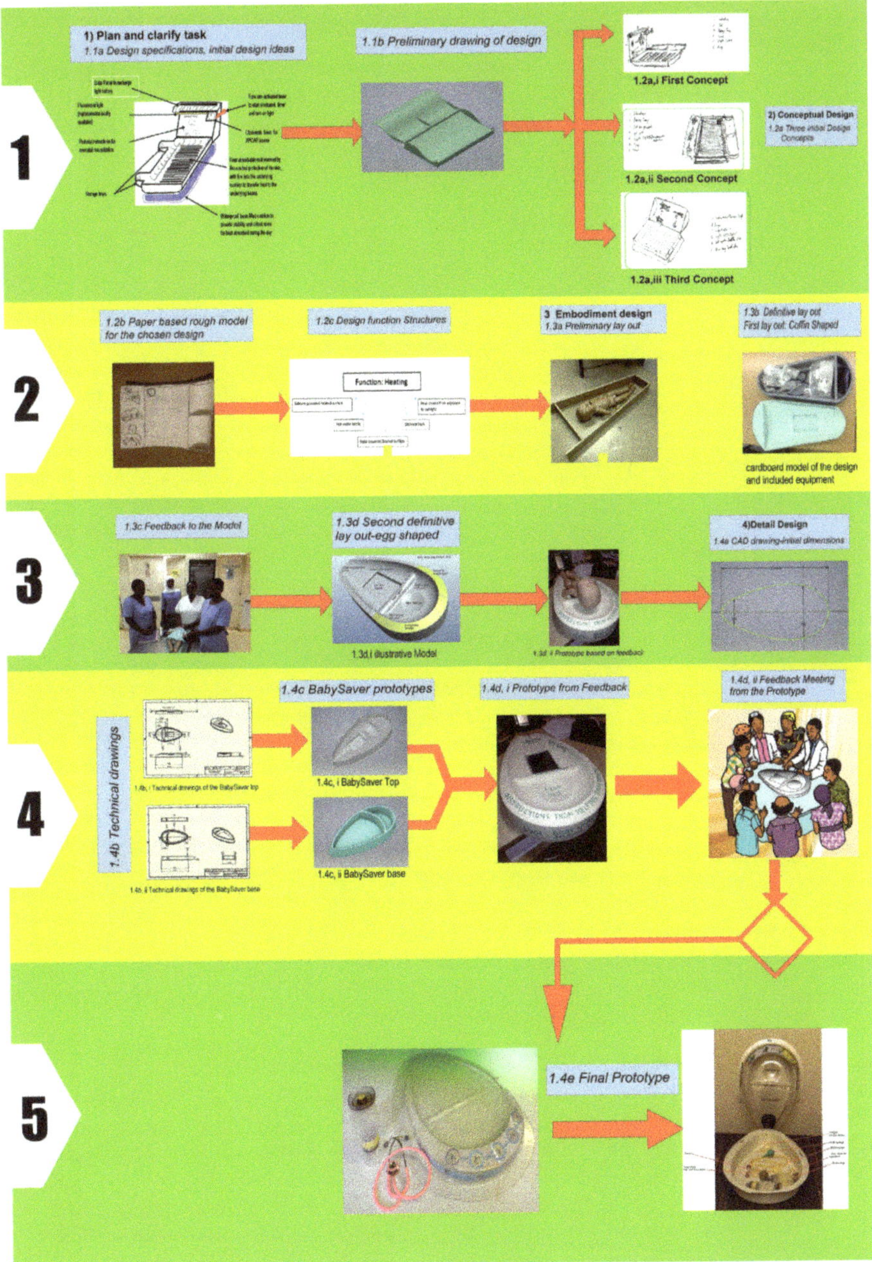

Figure 1. Steps in the planning and design process. (**1**). First phase, plan and clarify the task. (**2**). Second phase, the conceptual design. (**3**). Third phase, embodiment design. (**4**). Fourth phase, detailed design. (**5**). Outcome from all phases.

2.3. *Plan and Clarify the Task*

The development of the device was informed by the best practice reviews that recommend delayed cord clamping at birth [23–25], the experience of using the LifeStart trolley in the United Kingdom [14,15], and recommendations for promoting delayed cord clamping for transition at birth [26–28].

Though local guidelines in Uganda still recommend immediate cord clamping [29], many skilled birth attendants practice a degree of delayed cord clamping; an audit at Mbale regional referral hospital in 2016 found a median time to cord clamping of 87 s in vaginal births [30]. This meant that delayed cord clamping should not be difficult to implement if there could be a device to facilitate resuscitation at the mother's side.

2.3.1. Design Team Formation

In February 2015, a design team was formed, composed of Chris Dewhurst (consultant neonatologist), Julius Wandabwa (professor of obstetrics), Peter Watt (design engineer), James Ditai (research fellow), Julian Abeso (paediatrician), Bill Yoxall (consultant neonatologist), Sam Ononge (consultant obstetrician), Lelia Duley (professor of clinical trials) and Andrew Weeks (professor of international maternal health). A face-to-face meeting was held in the department of women's and children's health with some members of the design team, whilst others contributed virtually or through emailed comments. The meetings discussed resuscitation and cord clamping at birth in the delivery rooms of Uganda, design idea, initial design features, requirements, and constraints.

The design team proposed design specifications at this stage based on their experience, observation of the delivery environment, and informal consultation with staff of Mbale regional referral hospital in Uganda and LWH in the United Kingdom. Peter Watt and Aisling Barry, an MSc Engineering student, worked on the design process with further input from Nick Bettles (Inspiration Healthcare, Crawley, UK), Tony Fisher (professor and head of clinical engineering at Royal Liverpool University Hospital), Kathy Burgoine (neonatologist in Mbale), and Dot Lambert (research coordinator for the Sanyu Research Unit, University of Liverpool). Figure 1(1.1a) shows the initial design features. This resulted in an initial design that was used to seek funding.

2.3.2. Other Stakeholders

The design team enlisted the assistance of stakeholders who might interact with the device at different design phases in Uganda and the United Kingdom. These included end-users (women and their attendants, students of nursing, midwifery, and medicine, interns, a cleaner, midwives, nurses, medical officers, paediatricians, and obstetricians), developers (design and production engineers), regulatory authorities (the National Drugs Authority in Uganda, the Department of Medical Devices at the Ugandan Ministry of Health, and the Uganda National Council for Science and Technology), policymakers (the Ugandan Ministry of Health and the World Health Organization), and funders (Sir Halley Stewart, Grand Challenges Canada).

2.3.3. Problem Identification and Design Specification

The problems with the current method of resuscitation at birth were established through the personal experiences of the design team, ongoing consultation with relevant stakeholders, and observation of the delivery room facilities of Mulago National Referral Hospital and Mbale Regional Referral Hospital. Table 1 shows the resuscitation situational analysis carried out for Ugandan delivery environments. We modified the initial design specification to include what was desired from the new design (Table 2). We revised the design in line with the revised specification to produce the preliminary drawing in Figure 1(1.1b). A £14,300 funding proposal for the development of the modified design was submitted to the Sir Halley Stewart Trust and granted in October 2015.

Table 1. Situational analysis of resuscitation in labour and delivery suites in Uganda (2015).

S/No	Resuscitation Procedure in Delivery Rooms	Problems with the Current Method of Resuscitation at Birth	Mechanism of Action	Outcome
1	The baby is delivered by attending skilled birth attendant or student in the labour suite or operating theatre			
2	The baby's cord is clamped, or tied immediately and cut by the skilled birth attendant or student	Lack of a system to perform delayed cord clamping	Leads to decreased blood volume, haemoglobin and iron stores	An effect on baby's neurological development
3	The baby is dried and kept warm by the attending skilled birth attendant or student	Transfer of baby to a separate resuscitation station	Maternal-baby separation leading to fear of babies being swapped	Maternal distress
4	The baby is transferred to a resuscitaire/resuscitation station if it does not cry	Resuscitaire is not functional or broken	Resuscitation may be performed inadequately on available surfaces	Unnecessary death
5	The baby's airways are checked for any secretions and cleared if needed by wiping with a cloth or suctioning	Lack of constant electricity in delivery rooms	Absence of a heating option for the baby on the resuscitaire	Risk of hypothermia during resuscitation on the resuscitaire
6	The baby's back is rubbed 2−3 times, or feet slapped to stimulate breathing	Inconsistent or unavailable in-service training programme on helping babies breathe	Midwives not up to date with resuscitation guidelines or steps	Inability to follow guidelines for resuscitation
7	The baby is positioned in neutral position and ventilation initiated with bag and mask	Missing equipment for resuscitation	Inability to perform all the necessary steps of resuscitation	Unsuccessful resuscitation
8	If available, a mixture of oxygen and air is recommended for premature babies	Equipment is not in one place at time of resuscitation	Delays to initiate suctioning, bag and mask ventilation	Wasting of golden minute
9	If required after bag and mask ventilation, chest compressions are performed on the baby by a midwife			
10	If these are unsuccessful and drugs are available, drugs are administered by attending skilled birth attendant			
11	If resuscitation is successful, the baby is transferred to the neonatal unit			
12	The equipment used in the birth is taken for cleaning by the attending midwife	The equipment is cleaned in the same buckets as those for delivery		
13	The resuscitation equipment is maintained by the local engineering department			

Table 2. Design specification (the BabySaver wish list) in 2015.

S/No.	Requirement	Comments	Rank
1	The design must warm the baby to prevent hypothermia.	The heating should not harm the baby	1
2	The design must work with resuscitation protocols in place.	The systems may vary from hospital to hospital, but the tray should fit into standard practice in Mulago and Mbale hospitals	2
3	The design must be made of non-slip, cleanable materials.	The materials used must be able to be sterilised using current local cleaning practices	2
4	The design must provide pictorial instructions on how to deliver neonatal resuscitation.	This must agree with up-to-date standards of practice	3
5	The design must have storage capabilities for auxiliary equipment.		4
6	The design must be able to be moved safely.	This includes when in use	5
7	The design should be cheap to manufacture	Aim for manufacture price under $10	6
8	The design should have a light.	This should be independent from hospital utilities	7
9	The design should have a timer.		8
10	The design should be theft proof.	If possible, the design should discourage theft, or theft of parts.	9
11	The design should be able to be used on a variety of surfaces.		

2.4. Conceptual Design

2.4.1. Initial Design Concepts

The first concepts had a slatted surface to place the baby on, a solar-powered light, and a mechanical timer. The design was to be stored in the sun when not in use, and the resulting heat was stored in a solar-heated thermal capacitor (Figure 1(1.2a,i)).

The second concept was a box design with hinged flaps for storage and instructions, and a slot for a reusable heat gel pack to be inserted under the surface to diffuse heat throughout the design.

The heat gel pack was in a liquid state when inactive and solid form when active. The gel pack contained sodium acetate and water, activated by pressure on the inside metallic chip to generate heat through exothermic reaction to the design and inactivated under direct sunlight or boiling in the autoclave. The lights down each side of the design were for use at night or during maternity unit power cuts. They were intended to be powered by rechargeable batteries. The design folded easily for transport (Figure 1(1.2a,ii)).

In the third concept, a hot water bottle would be used for heat generation, and the heat stored in a bean bag base, which allowed the design to be placed on uneven surfaces, such as the mother's abdomen or legs. The lid functioned as both an equipment store and as a place to display the instructions (Figure 1(1.2a,iii)).

Choice of a Design Concept

Meetings were held with several stakeholders who evaluated the three designs and chose the second design. Their choice was based on its ease of use, replacement of parts, and infection control. The chosen design was seen as minimizing the space needed for resuscitation equipment and did not interfere with the practice of resuscitation. The heat gel pack was considered easy to maintain and could ensure the constant availability of the device. The solar-powered design would need to be always taken out for sunshine charging.

Heat Gel Pack

The feasibility of using a sunlight-activated heat gel pack for heat generation was tested in simple experiments. The used (solid) gel pack was exposed to the sunshine in Uganda to assess the time and ambient temperature required to melt it. Three hours of sun exposure at a maximum air temperature of 26.2 °C caused partial melting of the gel, but not to state where it could be reactivated. A second used gel pack was boiled in an autoclave at 103 °C for less than 5 min, wrapped in a linen cloth to prevent melting of the plastic shell of the gel pack against the metal. This led to the complete melting of the crystals.

Finally, questions about the use of the gel pack were raised in subsequent feedback meetings. Though both boiling and autoclaving could regenerate the gel pack, some users wanted to know if just pouring boiling water from a kettle over the pack would work instead, due to the common availability of kettles in the delivery suites. This indeed would melt the pack by direct boiling of the pack in the kettle with water.

Methods for Design Production

We explored two methods to produce the design; injection moulding (which was expensive and rejected) and thermoforming. Thermoforming is cheap, achieves less complicated shapes, and was subsequently chosen for mass production of the finished design [22].

Design Materials and Choices

Materials that were suitable for thermoforming were compared with the requirements for the design. The design needed to be made of a material that is strong, heat resistant, and that does not degrade when treated with bleach. The material of the device also needed to be biologically compatible. Consultation with a local plastics company ended in the recommendation to use Polyethylene terephthalate glycol-modified (PETG). PETG is a copolymerization of PET, which is a semicrystalline plastic. The addition of glycol prevents crystallization and lowers the melting temperature of the plastic.

2.4.2. Paper-Based Rough Design Model

PW made the first rough model out of hard paper and glue for the chosen design concept in 2015 (Figure 1(1.2b)).

2.4.3. Design Function Structures

Design solutions were generated with corresponding diagrams for each proposed device function or specification, using the brainstorming method. Figure 1(1.2c) shows an example of the design solutions and a diagram drawn for the heating function of the design. Other functions included storage, instruction display, light, and choice of materials.

Choice of Helping Babies Breathe (HBB) Instructions

The resuscitation instructions to be displayed on the design were chosen with the input of midwife Chiara Mosley, a neonatal resuscitation trainer from LWH. Initially, four stages of resuscitation had been recommended for displaying on the device, but later we choose to illustrate the key steps according to the HBB algorithm [31].

We initially planned to obtain permission from the HBB program to use their drawings as a pictorial illustration of instructions, but later produced our own. Two medical students (Bethany Harrison and Nathan Thompson) on elective placement designed the initial pictorial instructions, which were subsequently revised.

2.5. Embodiment Design

The stakeholders agreed with the purpose, content, scope, dimensions, and function of the design.

2.5.1. Preliminary Layout

Feedback Mbale Midwives

We sought feedback about the paper-based rough model from midwives in Mbale via group discussions in April 2015. The feedback included:

(i)   The rough model was not long enough for the baby and changes to the dimensions were proposed.

(ii)   The design required neck support as an add-in, to promote a natural neutral position during resuscitation.

(iii)   There were concerns that the timer could not sustain the bleaching effects of Sodium hypochlorite (Jik) solution following prolonged and frequent cleaning.

(iv)   They agreed with the need to include the storage tray for the pieces of equipment for resuscitation.

(v)   They proposed to add a valley on the top surface of the design as a slot for the gel pack. This would allow easier inserting and cleaning of the gel pack.

(vi)   Incorporating a light source in the tray would be incompatible with several specifications, especially "low cost and easy to sterilise using local methods".

(vii)   Light and timer were henceforth decided to be removed from the list and made as separate components to store in the design when needed.

Commonwealth and FIGO Fellows

We presented the modified design, alongside the rough design model, to the Commonwealth and FIGO Wellbeing Fellows (Fred Bisso, consultant ENT surgeon; Julian Abeso, paediatrician; Julius Wandabwa, obstetrician) in a meeting at the University Liverpool. They agreed with the proposed changes, one participant emphasizing that "even if the light and timer were separate or away for repair, the current design device could still be used". However, there was an argument against the neck support due to the different sizes of the baby and hence the need for different sizes of neck supports.

Positions of the Device at the Time of Resuscitation

Initially, the design was planned to be used on either the mother's abdomen or delivery bed. Stakeholders were concerned about the position of the maternal abdomen for the design at the time of resuscitation due to its weight and that of equipment. Further, the position of the abdomen and the side of the mother would not allow efficient blood transfer to the newborn by gravity. However, positioning the design in between the mother's legs on the delivery bed was considered appropriate to allow placental circulation with the umbilical cord intact. This generated an add-on design specification that ensures the baby is as close as possible to the mother. The design further had to assume a shape that fits in between the mother's legs in the lithotomy position. This formed the design for the preliminary layout.

Assembly of the Preliminary Layout

We took random measurements of the differently sized abdomen of gravid women and took the largest length and width for the design. Four pieces of timber were assembled to construct the design with narrow and broad ends. Figure 1(1.3a) shows the design in its preliminary layout with a model of the baby.

Cardboard Drawings

The team created a cardboard model showing the curve and dimensions of the preliminary layout, which was presented to midwives and obstetricians via face-to-face and international meetings. In these meetings, we sought feedback about the design and the process of use in a simulated labour environment from a lone midwife to a hospital team.

The feedback about the model in practical use helped identify the main areas of the design for remodelling.

2.5.2. First Version of Definitive Layout

We constructed a prototype following approval of the preliminary layout and materials. This was not a fully functional prototype, but a scale model made to demonstrate the functions and dimensions of the finished design.

The model was made from cardboard. Figure 1(1.3b) shows the design with the suggested contents. The sloped semicircle is where the picture of the resuscitation instructions would go.

Feedback on the First Version of Definitive Layout

The prototype was presented to 37 end users of Mulago national referral hospital and Mbale regional referral hospital, and two health centres in December 2015. These viewed the design as a device that could provide an additional location to resuscitate the baby without taking the midwife away from the delivery suite. However, the negative responses included the design's resemblance to a coffin, the unlikelihood of it fitting onto current beds, and dissatisfaction with current resuscitation practices. They recommended making the design's shape friendlier (less coffin-like), broadening one end and narrowing the curve at the other end. All agreed to the need for neck support but differed in opinion on its height. They proposed excluding the timer and providing multiple trays or coverings for sterile purposes. Figure 1(1.3c) shows the midwives in Mbale with the prototype in December 2016.

They suggested a clear tray to allow visibility of the pieces of equipment for resuscitation inside, child-friendly stickers, and more curves to the design. Several people requested that the tray be more ergonomically designed for resuscitation with a bag and mask, mostly centred on the rounding of the sharp edge where the curved section of the tray meets the instruction section. They also proposed making the base of the design flatter to look more like the weighing scales which are widely used. This was seen to have the added benefit of providing more room for the babies' shoulders.

Feedback on the Contents of the BabySaver Design

We sought feedback on the desired contents in the design. While most users were satisfied with the proposed auxiliary components, some wanted additional equipment. This ranged from thermometers to caps for babies, drugs, and cannulas. Though most people interviewed desired a timer to be included in the tray, they were happy with the current use of a wall clock for time.

However, it was subsequently argued that additional components would take focus away from the main key steps of resuscitation. Further, including consumables in the design would discourage use when they were gone or out of stock. We hence agreed to keep the main contents for resuscitation in the design. We hence classified contents into the design as essential and optional (Table 3).

Table 3. Equipment for resuscitation in the base of the BabySaver design.

Equipment and Supplies for the Care of Every Newborn at Birth in the BabySaver		
Essential equipment	Optional equipment	Optional Supplies
Suction device	NeoBeat newborn heart rate monitor	Surgical gloves
Neonatal Ambu Bag	Laryngoscope	Cord ties
Neonatal face mask size 1		Timer
Neonatal face mask size 0		Tetracycline eye ointment
Neonatal stethoscope		Vitamin K
		Intravenous fluids
		Adrenaline
		Oxytocin

2.5.3. Second Version of Definitive Layout

The definitive layout was proposed by Peter Watt and developed as part of the MSc engineering project for Aisling Barry. To escape the coffin shape, an egg shape was proposed, designed with more complex intersecting curves using Pro/Engineer 3D solid modelling software (Figure 1(1.3d,i)); and produced the first model using a computer numerical control (CNC) router in rigid modelling foam (Figure 1(1.3d,ii)).

Feedback on the Second Version of Definitive Layout

The egg-shaped 3D routed prototype in April 2017 was reviewed by paediatricians, obstetricians, doctors, and midwives in Uganda who all completed feedback sheets to comment on its design, shape, and functionality. This prototype was also reviewed by staff at the LWH neonatal intensive care unit (NICU), who provided written feedback. The final layout was achieved by December 2017.

2.6. Detailed Design

We produced the technical drawings of the version of the design to be made into the first functional prototype.

2.6.1. CAD Drawings

The revised design was drawn up using Autodesk Inventor, a computer-aided design software package. Figure 1(1.4a) shows a sample of the technical drawings of the final design.

2.6.2. Technical Drawings

Figure 1(1.4b) shows the sample technical drawings of the tray (i) and the base (ii). The drawings were done in a third-angle projection to ISO standards. All designs are intended for use with a 2 mm thick initial sheet of PET-G.

2.6.3. Prototype Initial Shape

Both the tray (Figure 1(1.4c,i)) and base (Figure 1(1.4c,ii)) for the initial shape of the design were constructed independently. The supporting walls of the base were hollow and set at a wide draft angle of 5 degrees to work better with the draw ratio constraints of thermoforming.

The top tray was constructed to fit snugly over the base, with 20 mm in between to provide passage for the users' fingers when lifting the top tray. The addition of the neck support and the increased smoothness of transitions between surfaces can be seen in the revised version of the design.

2.6.4. Feedback from Users in Uganda

We sought feedback in an interactive manner on the most recent version of the device (Figure 1(1.4d,i)) from women, health workers, and policymakers in Mbale regional referral hospital, Mulago national referral hospital, and the Ministry of Health. The following major changes were subsequently recommended.

The use of the gel packs was potentially troublesome; they could not be recharged rapidly or easily, there was a high chance of theft or damage, and there was a relatively high cost of replacement. We decided, therefore, to remove the gel packs, and hence a gel pack recess from the design in April 2017. This is shown in the final prototype manufactured for use in clinical testing, Figure 1(1.4e).

3. Results

3.1. Device Class

The device is a class I medical device [32] due to its transient, non-invasive, active therapeutic nature [33] and minimal risks established during the risk assessment for resuscitation [34] and COVID-19 [35]. Table 4 shows the risk assessment for the design.

Table 4. Risk assessment for the BabySaver design using a Failure mode and effects analysis (FMEA) form.

Key Process	Potential Failure Mode (FM)	Potential Failure Effects	SEV	Potential Causes	OCC	Current Controls	DET	RPN	Recommendations	Responsible Person
What is the process step or input?	In what ways can the process step or input fail?	What is the impact on the key output variables once it fails (customer or internal requirements)?	How severe is the effect on the customer?	What causes the key input to go wrong?	How often does cause or FM OCC occur?	What are the existing controls and procedures that prevent either the cause or the failure mode?	How well can you detect the cause or the failure mode?		What are the actions for reducing the occurrence of the cause, or improving detection?	Who is responsible for the recommended action?
Organise resuscitation equipment in the BabySaver	The bag and mask are non-functional	The baby receives inadequate ventilation	1	Defects in the pieces of equipment and limited user ability to detect early	1	All resuscitation equipment included in BabySaver should be checked before handing over to the hospital staff	1	4	User training	supplier/SAfRI/ Laerdal Global
BabySaver is brought close to the delivery bed	BabySaver falls	Midwife is injured	2	BabySaver held with slippery hands and in a rush	2	There is usually a delivery trolley in the labour suite, on which the BabySaver can be placed and moved	1	4	The users are trained on handling the BabySaver unit in a real clinical setting	Skilled birth attendant

Table 4. *Cont.*

Key Process	Potential Failure Mode (FM)	Potential Failure Effects	SEV	Potential Causes	OCC	Current Controls	DET	RPN	Recommendations	Responsible Person
Explain BabySaver to the mother and attendant	Mother scared of the device	Mother refuses the BabySaver use	2	Deliveries occurring before the explanation. Many deliveries under 1 midwife	2	All women are admitted to labour at a central station	1	4	Explanation of the device at any opportunity a midwife is in contact with the mother in labour during admission, examinations, etc.	Skilled birth attendant
Place the tray in between mother's legs	Tray slips	Mother and Baby are injured	2	A tray placed on an incompatible surface, no space in between legs. The tray is positioned wrongly with the broad end closet to the buttocks instead	2	Some delivery beds are long enough in the labour suite. For the surface material of the delivery beds, tests need to be performed to see how feasible this is.	1	4	User training on the positioning of the BabySaver, feasibility testing	Skilled birth attendant
Activates gel pack	The heat gel pack is not present	Baby's temperature drops	1	Equipment not replaced after use	3	The tray will have a checklist of equipment that should be included	1	3	Equipment included will be detailed in the instructions	Manufacturer

Table 4. *Cont.*

Key Process	Potential Failure Mode (FM)	Potential Failure Effects	SEV	Potential Causes	OCC	Current Controls	DET	RPN	Recommendations	Responsible Person
	Heat pack ruptures	Baby is injured	2	Heat pack has weak point due to incorrect care or manufacturing flaw	1	Pack contents non-toxic, pack contents not hot enough to injure	1	2	Instructions on pack care (not having the plastic on a hot surface, wrapping with a cloth while boiling, etc.) included	Manufacturer
	Heat pack overheats	Baby is injured	3	The pack is placed directly on neonate skin instead of through cloth	1	The heat gel pack has been tested to ensure it does not reach harmful heat levels	1	3	Instructions to regularly check the infant for erythema included	Manufacturer
	Heat pack underheats	Baby's temperature drops	1	Manufacturing error	1	Spare heat pack provided	2	2	Batch testing required	Manufacturer
Gently place the baby onto the tray	The baby is placed incorrectly	Resuscitation is incorrectly performed	1	Insufficient training	3	Neck support and pictorial instructions included	1	3	User training	Supplier/SAfRI/ manufacturer
Position the baby in a neutral position	The baby is positioned incorrectly	Resuscitation is incorrectly performed	1	The neck support is too elevated, or the neck support groove is too shallow	3	Minimum elevation of the neck support included	1	3	User training	Manufacturer

Table 4. *Cont.*

Key Process	Potential Failure Mode (FM)	Potential Failure Effects	SEV	Potential Causes	OCC	Current Controls	DET	RPN	Recommendations	Responsible Person
Keep the baby warm	The baby loses heat on the tray	Baby develops hypothermia	1	The baby is not covered in enough clothes, cotton dry clothes. Wet clothes not changed	3	The baby is dried and changed into a second warm cotton cloth before starting resuscitation	1	3	User training	Skilled birth attendant
Resuscitation is performed	Instructions are unclear	Resuscitation is incorrectly performed	3	Insufficient user training	1	Instructions are standard internationally agreed guidelines, checked with experienced practitioners for content.	2	6	User training, instructions also checked with inexperienced users for clarity	Supplier
	Tray fails mechanically	Mother and baby are injured	2	Too much force on the tray; sharp edges can cause discomfort	1	Durable material that does not degrade, smooth surface edges	2	4	Product lifecycle and surfaces of the edges advised in instructions	Manufacturer
	Mother kicks the tray during use	Midwife is injured	2	Maternal distress	1	Instructions for the user	2	4	User training and explaining to the mother early about the use of the BabySaver	Skilled birth attendant

Table 4. *Cont.*

Key Process	Potential Failure Mode (FM)	Potential Failure Effects	SEV	Potential Causes	OCC	Current Controls	DET	RPN	Recommendations	Responsible Person
Withdraw the tray from between mother's legs	The tray slips or is transferred to the ground	Midwife and mother injured	1	user oversight and fatigue, slippery gloves soiled in liquor and blood	3	The tray has a flat flap for firm handling	1	3	The users must be trained on proper handling of the tray with both hands where possible	Users/skilled birth attendants
Withdraw the equipment from the delivery field	Equipment is not replaced	Resuscitation is incorrectly performed	1	Replacement is not available, user oversight, pieces of equipment for resuscitation remain in mother's clothes	3	The tray has a checklist of equipment that should be included	1	3	Equipment included will be detailed on the instructions, as well as care instructions for the auxiliary components	Manufacturer
Reprocess the BabySaver and equipment	BabySaver is not disinfected fully	Baby contracts infection	2	Cleaning protocol not followed	3	The product has no crevasses; is compatible with local cleaning products	2	12	User training	Supplier

Table 4. *Cont.*

Key Process	Potential Failure Mode (FM)	Potential Failure Effects	SEV	Potential Causes	OCC	Current Controls	DET	RPN	Recommendations	Responsible Person
	BabySaver is not disinfected immediately	Baby contracts infection	2	Cleaning protocol not followed	3	The product has no crevasses; is compatible with local cleaning products	2	12	User training	Supplier
	Baby's pieces of equipment for resuscitation are mixed with maternal delivery pieces of equipment	Baby contracts infection	2	Cleaning protocol not followed	3	The product has no crevasses; is compatible with local cleaning products	2	12	User training	Supplier
The tray is returned to storage	Equipment is not replaced	Resuscitation is incorrectly performed	1	Replacement s not available, user oversight	3	The tray has a checklist of equipment that should be included	1	3	Equipment included will be detailed on the instructions, as well as care instructions for the auxiliary components	Manufacturer

SEV-Severity. OCC-Occurrence. DET-Detectability. RPN-Risk Prioritisation Number. FMEA-Failure Mode and Effects Analysis.

3.2. Device Description

The BabySaver is a simple, mobile, vacuum-moulded, and oval plastic assembly specifically designed to be used between the mother's legs or by the mother's side on the delivery bed. It provides a firm flat platform to resuscitate a depressed neonate at birth while the umbilical cord remains intact.

The weight of the developed design alone is 1850 g; the pieces of equipment for resuscitation weigh another 600 g. Figure 2 shows the final version of the BabySaver. Figure 3 shows its demonstration at birth with a model.

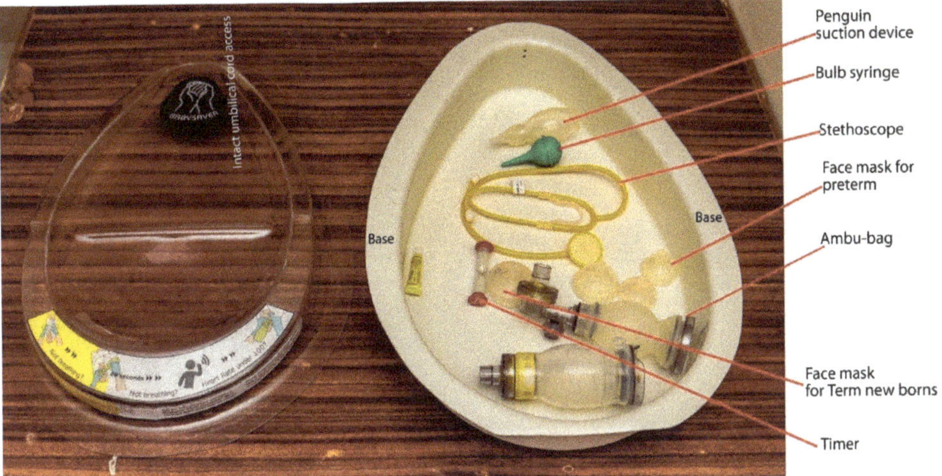

Figure 2. BabySaver design (current prototype). The BabySaver comprises two compartments: a tray at the top and a base at the bottom.

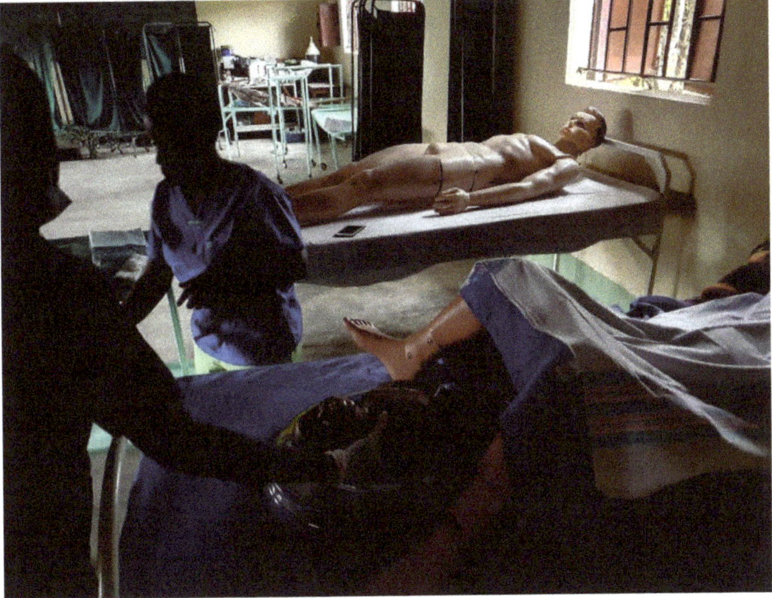

Figure 3. Demonstration of the BabySaver design at birth.

3.2.1. The Tray

The tray forms a clear plastic lid (Figure 4), that fits neatly into the base to form a toolbox. When the tray/lid is inverted, it forms a flat support platform. The platform provides a stable, clean, and smooth cradle to hold the neonate while the umbilical cord remains connected to the placenta at the time of birth. The weight of the tray is 950 g. The broad end is 455 mm wide, the longest length 685 mm and the depth 70 mm. It is 2 mm thick.

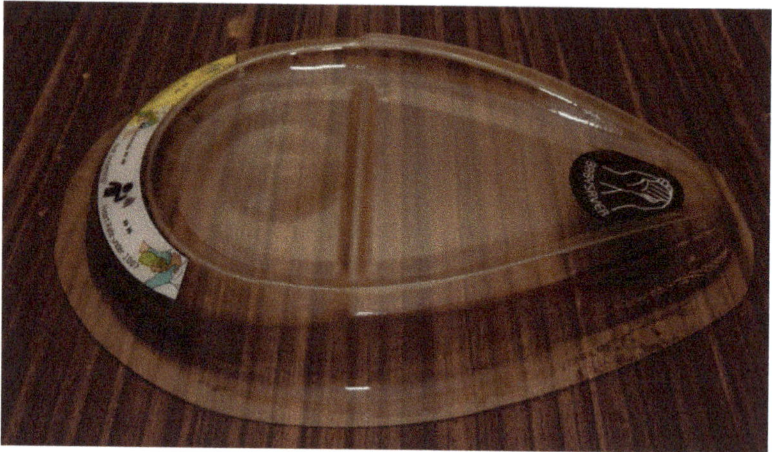

Figure 4. The tray.

The tray has a groove to receive and stabilise the baby's head. The groove is a few millimetres deep. The raised neck support slightly extends the baby's neck, positions the head into the groove, and keeps the neck in a neutral position with ease.

The tray has adhesive labels on its under surface which ensure that the top surface is completely smooth. The labels, visible through the plastic, carry icons and abbreviated instructions to act as a reminder for the skilled birth attendant (SBA) (Figure 5). These resuscitation instructions were adapted from the HBB programme [36], which is widely used in Uganda. It is easy to clean the tray.

3.2.2. The Base

The base is a non slip white plastic compartment. It has space for all the essential pieces of equipment for resuscitation at birth recommended for HBB [31] and the supplies necessary for essential newborn care for every baby at birth.

The base is specifically in white to easily detect any stain and is suitable for use on the resuscitation table, a delivery bed, an operation table, or any other available surface.

The weight of the base alone is 900 g. It is 103 mm deep with the widest broad end measuring 455 mm and its length is 685 mm. It is 3 mm thick, Figure 6.

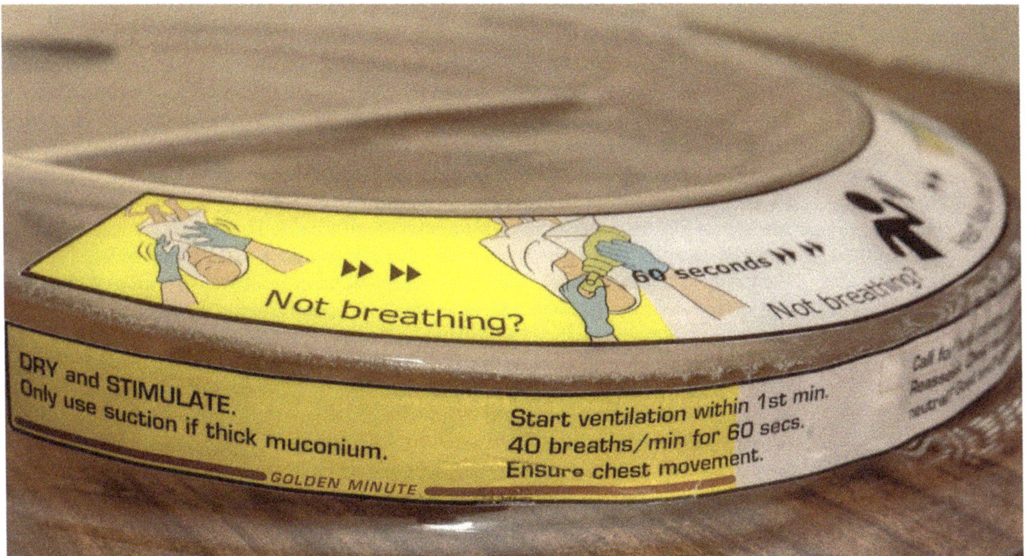

Figure 5. Pictorial instructions of helping babies breathe on the tray.

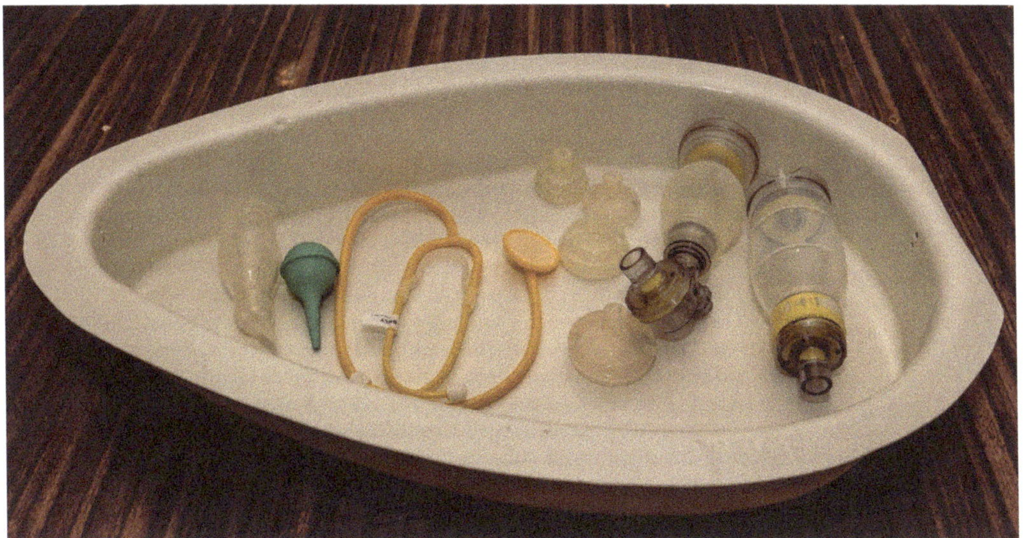

Figure 6. The base.

4. Discussion

Providing neonatal resuscitation at the bedside with an intact umbilical cord is potentially a high benefit practice with major global benefits [9–11]. The development of a low-cost and sustainable platform is central to this process. We have described the design process for a device that enables neonatal resuscitation with an intact umbilical cord without taking the midwife away from the mother's delivery bed [9–11]. This is the first device designed for use where there is a lone midwife on duty in the labour and delivery suite. This is a common occurrence in the developing world, where neonatal resuscitation

9.   Hutchon, D.; Bettles, N. Motherside care of the term neonate at birth. *Matern. Health Neonatol. Perinatol.* **2016**, *2*, 1–4. [CrossRef] [PubMed]
10.   Hutchon, D.; Pratesi, S.; Katheria, A. How to Provide Motherside Neonatal Resuscitation with Intact Placental Circulation? *Child* **2021**, *8*, 291. [CrossRef]
11.   Katheria, A.C.; Brown, M.K.; Rich, W.; Arnell, K. Providing a Placental Transfusion in Newborns Who Need Resuscitation. *Front. Pediatr.* **2017**, *5*, 1–8.
12.   Hutchon, D. Evolution of neonatal resuscitation with intact placental circulation. *Infant* **2014**, *10*, 58–61.
13.   Hutchon, D.J.R. Early versus delayed cord clamping at birth: In sickness and in health. *Fetal Matern. Med. Rev.* **2013**, *24*, 185–193. [CrossRef]
14.   Thomas, M.R.; Yoxall, C.W.; Weeks, A.D.; Duley, L. Providing newborn resuscitation at the mother's bedside: Assessing the safety, usability and acceptability of a mobile trolley. *BMC Pediatr.* **2014**, *14*, 135. [CrossRef]
15.   Weeks, A.; Watt, P.; Yoxall, C.W.; Gallagher, A.; Burleigh, A.; Bewley, S.; Heuchan, A.M.; Duley, L. Innovation in immediate neonatal care: Development of the Bedside Assessment, Stabilisation and Initial Cardiorespiratory Support (BASICS) trolley. *BMJ Innov.* **2015**, *1*, 53–58. [CrossRef] [PubMed]
16.   Brouwer, E.; Knol, R.; Vernooij, A.S.N.; Akker, T.V.D.; Vlasman, P.E.; Klumper, F.J.C.M.; Dekoninck, P.; Polglase, G.R.; Hooper, S.B.; Pas, A.B.T. Physiological-based cord clamping in preterm infants using a new purpose-built resuscitation table: A feasibility study. *Arch. Dis. Child. Fetal Neonatal Ed.* **2018**, *104*, F396–F402. [CrossRef] [PubMed]
17.   Knol, R.; Brouwer, E.; Vernooij, A.S.N.; Klumper, F.J.C.M.; Dekoninck, P.; Hooper, S.B.; Pas, A.B.T. Clinical aspects of incorporating cord clamping into stabilisation of preterm infants. *Arch. Dis. Child. Fetal Neonatal Ed.* **2018**, *103*, F493–F497. [CrossRef]
18.   Knol, R.; Brouwer, E.; Akker, T.V.D.; DeKoninck, P.; van Geloven, N.; Polglase, G.R.; Lopriore, E.; Herkert, E.; Reiss, I.K.; Hooper, S.B.; et al. Physiological-based cord clamping in very preterm infants Randomised controlled trial on effectiveness of stabilisation. *Resuscitation* **2020**, *147*, 26–33. [CrossRef]
19.   Knol, R.; Brouwer, E.; Klumper, F.J.C.M.; Akker, T.V.D.; Dekoninck, P.; Hutten, G.J.; Lopriore, E.; Van Kaam, A.H.; Polglase, G.R.; Reiss, I.K.M.; et al. Effectiveness of Stabilization of Preterm Infants with Intact Umbilical Cord Using a Purpose-Built Resuscitation Table—Study Protocol for a Randomized Controlled Trial. *Front. Pediatr.* **2019**, *7*, 134. [CrossRef] [PubMed]
20.   Katheria, A.; Lee, H.C.; Knol, R.; Irvine, L.; Thomas, S. A review of different resuscitation platforms during delayed cord clamping. *J. Perinatol.* **2021**, *13*, 1–9.
21.   Niermeyer, S.; Robertson, N.J.; Ersdal, H.L. Beyond basic resuscitation: What are the next steps to improve the outcomes of resuscitation at birth when resources are limited? *Semin. Fetal Neonatal Med.* **2018**, *23*, 361–368. [CrossRef]
22.   Pahl, G.; Beitz, W.; Feldhusen, J.; Grote, K.-H. *Engineering Design: A Systematic Approach*, 3rd ed.; Springer: London, UK, 2007.
23.   Fogarty, M.; Osborn, D.A.; Askie, L.; Seidler, A.L.; Hunter, K.; Lui, K.; Simes, J.; Tarnow-Mordi, W. Delayed vs. early umbilical cord clamping for preterm infants: A systematic review and meta-analysis. *Am. J. Obstet. Gynecol.* **2018**, *218*, 1–18. [CrossRef]
24.   Rabe, H.; Gyte, G.M.; Díaz-Rossello, J.L.; Duley, L. Effect of timing of umbilical cord clamping and other strategies to influence placental transfusion at preterm birth on maternal and infant outcomes. *Cochrane Database Syst. Rev.* **2019**, *9*, CD003248. [CrossRef]
25.   Rabe, H.; Reynolds, G.J.; Diaz-Rosello, J.L. Early versus delayed umbilical cord clamping in preterm infants. *Cochrane Database Syst. Rev.* **2004**, *77*, CD003248. [CrossRef]
26.   Matar, H.E.; Almerie, M.Q.; Alsabbagh, M.; Jawoosh, M.; Almerie, Y.; Abdulsalam, A.; Duley, L. Policies for care during the third stage of labour: A survey of maternity units in Syria. *BMC Pregnancy Childbirth* **2010**, *10*, 32. [CrossRef]
27.   Madar, J.; Roehr, C.C.; Ainsworth, S.; Ersdal, H.; Morley, C.; Rüdiger, M.; Skåre, C.; Szczapa, T.; Pas, A.T.; Trevisanuto, D.; et al. European Resuscitation Council Guidelines 2021: Newborn resuscitation and support of transition of infants at birth. *Resuscitation* **2021**, *161*, 291–326. [CrossRef]
28.   World Health Organisation. *Guideline: Delayed Umbilical Cord Clamping for Improved Maternal and Infant Health and Nutrition Outcomes*; WHO: Geneva, Switzerland, 2014.
29.   Ministry of Health. *Uganda Clinical Guidelines 2016: National Guidelines for Management of Common Conditions, Revised*; Ministry of Health Uganda: Kampala, Uganda, 2016.
30.   Mitchell, E.J.; Benjamin, S.; Ononge, S.; Ditai, J.; Qureshi, Z.; Masood, S.N.; Whitham, D.; Godolphin, P.J.; Duley, L. Identifying women giving birth preterm and care at the time of birth: A prospective audit of births at six hospitals in India, Kenya, Pakistan and Uganda. *BMC Pregnancy Childbirth* **2020**, *20*, 1–10. [CrossRef] [PubMed]
31.   Niermeyer, S. From the Neonatal Resuscitation Program to Helping Babies Breathe: Global impact of educational programs in neonatal resuscitation. *Semin. Fetal Neonatal Med.* **2015**, *20*, 300–308. [CrossRef] [PubMed]
32.   Ogrodnik, P.J. *Class 1 Devices: Case Studies in Medical Devices Design*; Elsevier: London, UK, 2015.
33.   Soth, M.; Piraino, T. *Noninvasive Mechanical Ventilation: Theory, Equipment, and Clinical Applications, Second*; Springer International Publishing: New York, NY, USA, 2016.
34.   Madar, J. Clinical risk management in newborn and neonatal resuscitation. *Semin. Fetal Neonatal Med.* **2005**, *10*, 45–61. [CrossRef]
35.   Uganda National Council for Science and Technology (UNCST). *National Guidelines for Conduct of Research during Corona Virus Disease 2019 (COVID-19) Pandemic, July*; Uganda National Council for Science and Technology: Kampala, Uganda, 2020.
36.   Bang, A.; Bellad, R.; Gisore, P.; Hibberd, P.; Patel, A.; Goudar, S.; Esamai, F.; Goco, N.; Meleth, S.; Derman, R.J.; et al. Implementation and evaluation of the Helping Babies Breathe curriculum in three resource limited settings: Does Helping Babies Breathe save lives? A study protocol. *BMC Pregnancy Childbirth* **2014**, *14*, 116. [CrossRef]

37. Kamath-Rayne, B.D.; Thukral, A.; Visick, M.K.; Schoen, E.; Amick, E.; Deorari, A.; Cain, C.J.; Keenan, W.J.; Singhal, N.; Little, G.A.; et al. Helping Babies Breathe, Second Edition: A Model for Strengthening Educational Programs to Increase Global Newborn Survival. *Glob. Health Sci. Pract.* **2018**, *6*, 538–551. [CrossRef]

38. Singhal, N.; Lockyer, J.; Fidler, H.; Keenan, W.; Little, G.; Bucher, S.; Qadir, M.; Niermeyer, S. Helping Babies Breathe: Global neonatal resuscitation program development and formative educational evaluation. *Resuscitation* **2012**, *83*, 90–96. [CrossRef] [PubMed]

39. Mann, C.; Chilcott, S.; Plumb, K.; Brooks, E.; Man, M.-S. Reporting and appraising the context, process and impact of PPI on contributors, researchers and the trial during a randomised controlled trial—the 3D study. *Res. Involv. Engag.* **2018**, *4*, 1–12. [CrossRef] [PubMed]

40. INVOLVE. *Public Involvement in Clinical Trials: Supplement to the Briefing Notes for Researchers*; Eastleigh: Hampshire, UK, 2012.

41. Martin, J.L.; Murphy, E.; Crowe, J.; Norris, B.J. Capturing user requirements in medical device development: The role of ergonomics. *Physiol. Meas.* **2006**, *27*, R49–R62. [CrossRef] [PubMed]

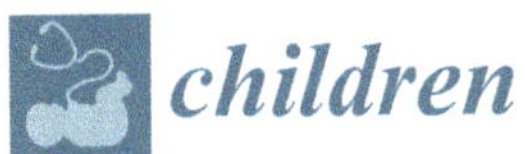

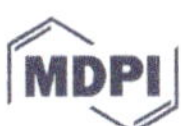

Brief Report

A Feasibility Study of a Novel Delayed Cord Clamping Cart

Neha S. Joshi [1,*], Kimber Padua [1], Jules Sherman [2], Douglas Schwandt [1], Lillian Sie [1], Arun Gupta [1], Louis P. Halamek [1] and Henry C. Lee [1,*]

1   Department of Pediatrics, Stanford University, Stanford, CA 94305, USA; kpadua@stanford.edu (K.P.); doug.schwandt@gmail.com (D.S.); lillsie@stanford.edu (L.S.); agup@stanford.edu (A.G.); halamek@stanford.edu (L.P.H.)
2   The Hasso Plattner Institute of Design, Stanford University, Stanford, CA 94305, USA; julessherman@alumni.stanford.edu
*   Correspondence: nsjoshi@stanford.edu (N.S.J.); hclee@stanford.edu (H.C.L.)

Abstract: Delaying umbilical cord clamping (DCC) for 1 min or longer following a neonate's birth has now been recommended for preterm and term newborns by multiple professional organizations. DCC has been shown to decrease rates of iron deficiency anemia, intraventricular hemorrhage (IVH), necrotizing enterocolitis (NEC), and blood transfusion. Despite these benefits, clinicians typically cut the umbilical cord without delay in neonates requiring resuscitation and move them to a radiant warmer for further care; this effectively prevents these patients from receiving any benefits from DCC. This study evaluated the feasibility of a delayed cord clamping cart (DCCC) in low-risk neonates born via Cesarean section (CS). The DCCC is a small, sterile cart designed to facilitate neonatal resuscitation while the umbilical cord remains intact. The cart is cantilevered over the operating room (OR) table during a CS, allowing the patient to be placed onto it immediately after birth. For this study, a sample of 20 low-risk CS cases were chosen from the non-emergency Labor and Delivery surgical case list. The DCCC was utilized for 1 min of DCC in all neonates. The data collected included direct observation by research team members, recorded debriefings and surveys of clinicians as well as surveys of patients. Forty-four care team members participated in written surveys; of these, 16 (36%) were very satisfied, 12 (27%) satisfied, 13 (30%) neutral, and 3 (7%) were somewhat dissatisfied with use of the DCCC in the OR. Feedback was collected from all 20 patients, with 18 (90%) reporting that they felt safe with the device in use. This study provides support that utilizing a DCCC can facilitate DCC with an intact umbilical cord.

Keywords: neonatology; resuscitation; delayed cord clamping; simulation

Citation: Joshi, N.S.; Padua, K.; Sherman, J.; Schwandt, D.; Sie, L.; Gupta, A.; Halamek, L.P.; Lee, H.C. A Feasibility Study of a Novel Delayed Cord Clamping Cart. *Children* **2021**, *8*, 357. https://doi.org/10.3390/children8050357

Academic Editor: Simone Pratesi

Received: 16 April 2021
Accepted: 27 April 2021
Published: 29 April 2021

Publisher's Note: MDPI stays neutral with regard to jurisdictional claims in published maps and institutional affiliations.

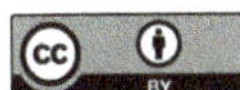

1. Introduction

Delayed cord clamping (DCC) refers to the practice of delaying clamping of a neonate's umbilical cord for at least 30–60 s after birth. This delay in clamping of the umbilical cord effectively allows for a blood transfusion from the placental bed into the newborn's circulation [1–5]. Studies suggest that 75% of available blood in the placenta is transfused to the infant within 1 min [6]. DCC has noted benefits in both preterm and term neonates. In preterm neonates, DCC is associated with increased hematocrit levels, decreased need for blood transfusion, and decreased incidence of NEC and IVH [7–9]. Term neonates receiving DCC have increased hemoglobin levels at birth, increased iron stores at 6 months of age, and potentially improved neurodevelopmental outcomes [6–10]. Given its known benefits, DCC has been endorsed by multiple professional organizations, including the World Health Organization, the International Liaison Committee on Resuscitation, the American Academy of Pediatrics, and the American College of Obstetricians and Gynecologists, amongst several others [1–5,11]. These professional organizations recommend DCC in most vigorous preterm and term neonates.

Some reasons for not performing DCC include the need for immediate neonatal resuscitation, maternal bleeding, and concern for an intact maternal-neonatal umbilical cord circulation. Neonates requiring immediate resuscitation often receive immediate cord clamping due to the challenging ergonomics of performing resuscitation during DCC. Following cord clamping, these patients are carried to a radiant warmer provisioned with resuscitation equipment and supplies such as oxygen, suctioning, and positive pressure ventilation capability.

Providing continuous positive airway pressure (CPAP) immediately at birth to premature neonates born at <28 weeks gestational age reduces the need for respiratory interventions such as exogenous surfactant administration and mechanical ventilation while potentially reducing the severity of respiratory distress syndrome and incidence of bronchopulmonary dysplasia [12,13]. Presently, it is not practical in most circumstances for neonates to receive both immediate CPAP or other forms of neonatal resuscitation, and also receive DCC, given the logistical difficulties of current standard hospital equipment.

To address the logistical challenges of providing resuscitation including CPAP or positive pressure ventilation during DCC, our team designed a sterile compact cart (the Delayed Cord Clamping Cart, DCCC) that can be positioned near the incision site during a CS or by a mother's bedside during a vaginal delivery, allowing for resuscitation to be performed during DCC. We conducted a study in order to evaluate the feasibility of using this DCCC during CS deliveries.

2. Materials and Methods

2.1. Cart Design

Our research team had previously performed simulations and debriefings of childbirth focusing on DCC while resuscitating the infant [14]. Based on this work, the team designed and prototyped a cart to facilitate DCC while allowing for the possibility of simultaneous respiratory support (Figure 1). Iterations of the prototype occurred based on further repeated simulations involving a multidisciplinary team at the Stanford Medicine Center for Advanced Pediatric and Perinatal Education (CAPE, http://cape.stanford.edu, accessed on 28 April 2021). The development of the DCCC began with simple concept sketches, and subsequently evolved to increasingly more complex functional models using SolidWorks Premium 2021 computer aided design (CAD) software. These models focused on planning the mechanical structure, mechanisms, and electrical features of the cart.

For stability purposes, it was essential for the DCCC cart base to have sufficient floor support in addition to the ballast required to counterweight the extension of the tray well beyond the wheeled base. Initially, simple support blades similar to those found on traditional Mayo stands, were trialed to minimize tipping of the DCCC. These were subsequently updated to utilizing castering wheels, in order to maximize easy mobility of the DCCC. An intravenous pole was placed in the back with the requisite resuscitation equipment. Air and oxygen cylinders were strategically placed at the base of the intravenous pole to help generate sufficient ballast for extending the resuscitation tray forward to allow it to safely cantilever over the operating table. Tipping analyses were performed, taking into account dynamic movement of the cart.

A single telescoping column was placed at the front of the cart to provide approximately 65 cm (25.6 in) of vertical adjustment, allowing the tray to be adjusted from about 68 to 133 cm (26.8 to 52.3 in) height above the floor. The DCCC's arm extends from a proximal rotary joint at the top of the column to another distal rotary joint below the tray. A prismatic sliding joint under the tray provides additional reach. The telescoping column combined with the rotary and prismatic joints allow for flexibility in both positioning and orientation of the tray to make it easier to safely place the neonate onto the DCCC tray without putting excessive traction on the neonate's umbilical cord.

A fully functional version of the DCCC incorporating these features was designed and fabricated. Simulations of the DCCC were conducted, with feedback received from the multidisciplinary working group. Once shown to be safe and effective during simulated deliveries, the DCCC was approved for use by the Biomedical Engineering Department at Lucile Packard Children's Hospital Stanford and this study was authorized by the Institutional Review Board (IRB) of Stanford University.

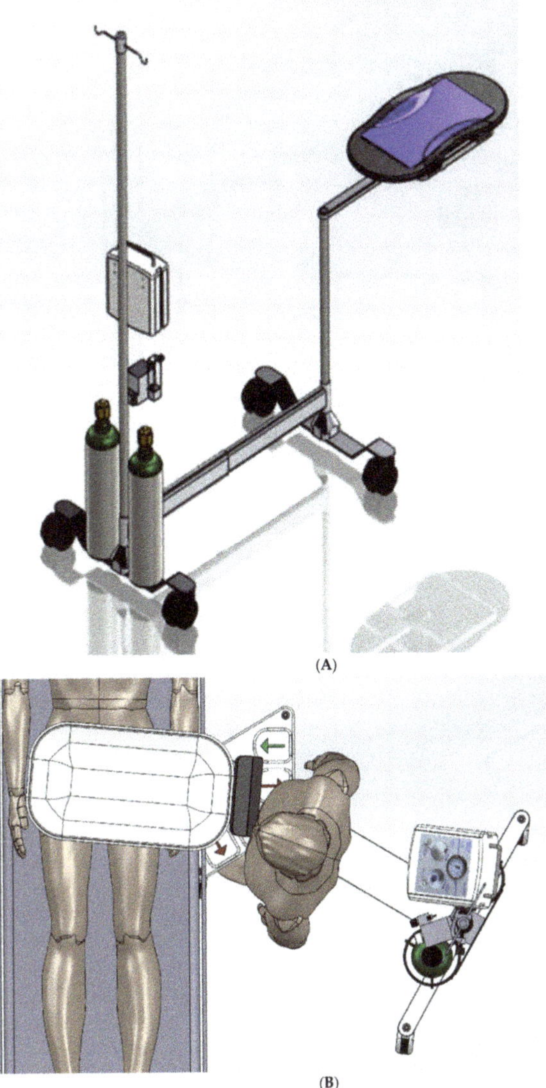

(A)

(B)

Figure 1. (**A**) Schematic rendering of delayed cord clamping cart. (**B**) Schematic rendering of delayed cord clamping cart cantilevered over patient's abdomen during CS.

The DCCC is a small, mobile sterile cart (Figures 1 and 2) designed to facilitate resuscitation while the umbilical cord is intact. The DCCC is designed to cantilever, extending from the cart over the operating room (OR) table during a CS, allowing for the newborn to be placed directly onto it immediately at the time of birth. As described above, the DCCC is equipped with mechanisms that facilitate vertical movement, positioning and orientation over the OR table, and wheels for maneuverability around the room. It is designed to accommodate the equipment used during neonatal resuscitation.

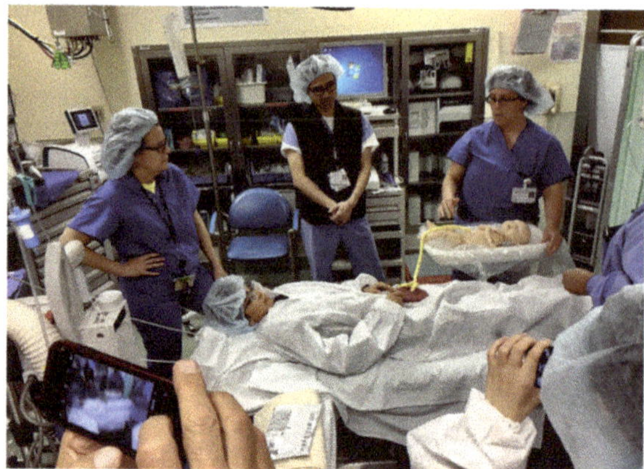

Figure 2. Delayed cord clamping cart in use during a simulation.

2.2. Study

A sample of 20 scheduled low-risk CS cases were chosen to pilot the DCCC. Written informed consent was obtained from patients and the members of the multidisciplinary OR team (pediatricians, obstetricians, anesthesiologists, nursing staff, and surgical technicians). Each multidisciplinary team member was trained in the use of the DCCC.

In this observational study, a research team member observed the use of the DCCC and its effectiveness in facilitating DCC during CS. Without the DCCC, the standard procedure includes placing the neonate on the mother's abdomen or having a clinician hold the neonate during DCC. With the DCCC, the neonate was placed directly onto the cart at the time of delivery. Once the cord was clamped, the patient was moved to the radiant warmer while remaining on the DCCC, then transitioned to the radiant warmer for further evaluation and care. Otherwise, the cart did not influence or change the current provider procedures in the operating room. Video recordings of the procedure were made, and structured interviews and written surveys of all team members were conducted after the CS. Written surveys were completed by patients after recovery.

The primary end-point was to evaluate the safety and efficacy of the DCCC. Immediately following each case, the clinicians were asked to participate in a structured interview about their experience using the DCCC and to identify any elements of the cart that could be improved. Patients and their partners were given a short survey 12–24 h postpartum regarding their experience with the DCCC.

2.3. Data Analysis

The data presented here reflect approximately 20 h of observation. Demographic data were analyzed using counts and percentages. The structured interviews from patients and providers were transcribed and analyzed for thematic patterns. Once recurring themes from the analyses were identified, the research team made improvements to the cart accordingly. The surveys from the patients were analyzed and triaged for patient safety and patient experience.

3. Results

The DCCC was used in 20 CS deliveries of term singletons from October 2018 to January 2020. Gestational age at the time of delivery ranged from 36 to 39 weeks. Enrolled patients were pre-identified as low risk for anticipated maternal and neonatal complications at the time of delivery by the delivering obstetrician. All neonates were vigorous at delivery, and received 60 s of DCC on the DCCC; no neonates required resuscitation.

There were 159 providers who participated in the CS that utilized the DCCC. The multidisciplinary team members directly interacting with the cart included attending neonatal hospitalists, pediatric resident physicians, attending obstetricians, obstetrician resident physicians, and obstetric surgical technicians. Neonatal nurses, obstetric nurses, and members of the anesthesia team were included in the informed consent process but did not directly interact with the cart; formal interviews and written feedback was not collected from those not directly interacting with the cart given that the DCCC neither supported nor impeded their workflow.

Data collected from structured interviews of team members and patients reflects approximately 20 h of recordings, which were transcribed and subsequently analyzed. Forty-four care team members participated in written surveys. Sixteen providers (36%) were very satisfied, 12 (27%) satisfied, 13 (30%) neutral, and 3 (7%) were somewhat dissatisfied with use of the DCCC in the OR. Team members commented that the cart was easily incorporated into the surgical field without concern for breaking sterility, and was not a hindrance during the surgery. An obstetrician noted that the usage of the DCCC "improved baby positioning" compared to without the cart, and another noted that the DCCC "just seems more stable" for the neonate. Given that umbilical cords vary in length, team members noted the need for close evaluation and adjustment in positioning of the DCCC to prevent excessive traction on the cord during DCC. The most frequently noted concern involved maneuvering the cart from the OR table to the radiant warmer. No adverse safety events occurred to either the mother or infant during any of the CS trials with the DCCC.

Feedback was additionally collected from 18 patients, with 2 patients lost to follow up. Seventeen patients (94%) reported that it was easy to communicate with the hospital staff while the device was in use; one patient (5%) felt neutral. Eighteen patients (100%) reported they felt safe when the device was in use. No adverse outcomes for mothers or neonates were noted.

Video recordings of all 20 CS deliveries were watched by the research team. Recurring themes noticed on video recordings and in team member surveys were employed to update the features of the DCCC. These changes included adjustments in the height of the cart's tray side walls for more secure positioning during the cart's usage, and adding hand switches under the tray similar to existing foot manual controls to allow for two ways to adjust the DCCC's height for each delivery.

4. Discussion

Facilitating successful DCC has several benefits for both preterm and term neonates. While DCC is now standard of care in vigorous newborns, it is likely that non-vigorous patients requiring resuscitation may also benefit from DCC. Studies in lambs have shown that DCC while the animal establishes ventilation confers hemodynamic stability during the transition to the extrauterine environment [15]. Aeration of the lungs during spontaneous ventilation triggers pulmonary vasodilation and an increase in pulmonary blood flow; this increased pulmonary blood flow then provides critical preload to the left ventricle and supports systemic perfusion and blood pressure [16]. DCC, through its transfusion of placental blood into the neonatal circulation and subsequent increase in left ventricular preload, can thus confer hemodynamic stability to vigorous preterm and term neonates, and may also benefit those who are non-vigorous at birth if they are receiving positive pressure ventilation. Facilitating DCC while allowing for the beginning steps of neonatal resuscitation to take place is especially beneficial in preterm infants, who are at highest need for neonatal resuscitation and also likely stand to benefit the most from DCC's protective effects.

A mobile cart to facilitate DCC has been previously described in the literature and work continues to refine design and standardize equipment [17–19]. There are currently two such carts that are commercially available: the Life Start® Trolley [West Sussex, United Kingdom] and the INSPiRe Platform. However, neither of these devices are specifically designed to get close enough to the mother's incision site so that a preterm neonate can remain attached to the umbilical cord while CPAP is being performed. In clinical trials, these devices could not be used in 30% of deliveries due to their bulky design [20,21].

We evaluated the ergonomics and feasibility of a sterile DCCC to be utilized during CS and vaginal deliveries in order to enable resuscitation with an intact cord. Given its goals, 20 low-risk CS deliveries in term neonates were selected for inclusion; none of these neonates required resuscitation. The DCCC received overall favorable feedback from team members regarding ease of use. All patients reported that they felt safe during use of the DCCC with their newborns and most noted that they were able to communicate easily with their care team during the DCCC's usage. Team members often commented on the ease with which the DCCC incorporated into the existing workflow for CS deliveries, which is key to allowing for successful adaptation and implementation of the cart. A limitation of this study is its utilization in only a relatively small number of low-risk CS deliveries of infants not requiring resuscitation; however, data obtained from this study will be used to further refine the DCCC for studies to determine its safety, efficacy, and feasibility in vaginal deliveries and in preterm and term neonates requiring resuscitation at birth. Further studies utilizing the DCCC could additionally capture clinical outcomes of neonatal resuscitation. In summary, our study provides support that the DCCC can facilitate DCC in vigorous term neonates while the umbilical cord remains intact.

Author Contributions: Conceptualization, N.S.J., J.S., D.S., L.S., H.C.L.; methodology, formal analysis, investigation, data curation: all authors; writing—original draft preparation, N.S.J.; writing—review and editing, K.P., J.S., D.S., L.S., A.G., L.P.H., H.C.L.; supervision, H.C.L. All authors have read and agreed to the published version of the manuscript.

Funding: This study was funded by Agency for Healthcare Research and Quality (Grant/Award Number: 'P30HS023506') and the Maternal and Child Health Research Institute at Stanford University.

Institutional Review Board Statement: The Delayed Cord Clamping Cart was approved for use by the Biomedical Engineering Department at Lucile Packard Children's Hospital Stanford and this study was authorized by the Institutional Review Board of Stanford University.

Informed Consent Statement: Informed consent was obtained from all subjects involved in the study.

Data Availability Statement: The data presented in this study are available on request from the corresponding author. The data are not publicly available due to privacy concerns.

Conflicts of Interest: The authors declare no conflict of interest. The funders had no role in the design of the study; in the collection, analyses, or interpretation of data; in the writing of the manuscript, or in the decision to publish the results.

References

1. World Health Organization. *Guideline: Delayed Umbilical Cord Clamping for Improved Maternal and Infant Health and Nutrition Outcomes*; World Health Organization: Geneva, Switzerland, 2014.
2. World Health Organization. *Guidelines on Basic Newborn Resuscitation*; World Health Organization: Geneva, Switzerland, 2012.
3. Wyckoff, M.H.; Aziz, K.; Escobedo, M.B.; Kapadia, V.S.; Kattwinkel, J.; Perlman, J.M.; Simon, W.M.; Weiner, G.M.; Zaichkin, J.G. Part 13: Neonatal Resuscitation: 2015 American Heart Association Guidelines Update for Cardiopulmonary Resuscitation and Emergency Cardiovascular Care. *Circulation* **2015**, *132* (Suppl. 2), S543–S560. [CrossRef] [PubMed]
4. Committee Opinion No. 543: Timing of Umbilical Cord Clamping After Birth. *Obstet. Gynecol.* **2012**, *120*, 1522–1526. [CrossRef] [PubMed]
5. Committee Opinion No. 684: Delayed Umbilical Cord Clamping After Birth. *Obs. Gynecol* **2017**, *129*, 1. [CrossRef]
6. Katheria, A.C.; Lakshminrusimha, S.; Rabe, H.; McAdams, R.; Mercer, J.S. Placental transfusion: A review. *J. Perinatol.* **2017**, *37*, 105–111. [CrossRef] [PubMed]
7. McDonald, S.J.; Middleton, P.; Dowswell, T.; Morris, P.S. Effect of timing of umbilical cord clamping of term infants on maternal and neonatal outcomes. *Evid. Based Child Health Cochrane Rev. J.* **2014**, *9*, 303–397. [CrossRef] [PubMed]
8. Lainez Villabona, B.; Bergel Ayllon, E.; Cafferata Thompson, M.L.; Belizán Chiesa, J.M. Early or late umbilical cord clamping? A systematic review of the literature. *Pediatria* **2005**, *63*, 14–21. [CrossRef]
9. Katheria, A.; Reister, F.; Essers, J.; Mendler, M.; Hummler, H.; Subramaniam, A.; Carlo, W.; Tita, A.; Truong, G.; Davis-Nelson, S.; et al. Association of Umbilical Cord Milking vs Delayed Umbilical Cord Clamping with Death or Severe Intraventricular Hemorrhage Among Preterm Infants. *JAMA* **2019**, *322*, 1877–1886. [CrossRef] [PubMed]

10. Isacson, M.; Gurung, R.; Basnet, O.; Andersson, O.; Kc, A. Neurodevelopmental outcomes of a randomised trial of intact cord resuscitation. *Acta Paediatr.* **2021**, *110*, 465–472. [CrossRef] [PubMed]
11. Weiner, G.; Zaichkin, J.G. *Textbook of Neonatal Resuscitation (NRP)*; American Academy of Pediatrics: Itasca, IL, USA, 2006.
12. Newborn, C.F.A. Respiratory Support in Preterm Infants at Birth. *Pediatrics* **2014**, *133*, 171–174. [CrossRef] [PubMed]
13. Dunn, M.S.; Kaempf, J.; de Klerk, A.; de Klerk, R.; Reilly, M.; Howard, D.; Ferrelli, K.; O'Conor, J.; Soll, R.F.; The Vermont Oxford Network DRM Study Group. Randomized Trial Comparing 3 Approaches to the Initial Respiratory Management of Preterm Neonates. *Pediatrics* **2011**, *128*, e1069–e1076. [CrossRef] [PubMed]
14. Lapcharoensap, W.; Cong, A.; Sherman, J.; Schwandt, D.; Crowe, S.; Daniels, K.; Lee, H.C. Safety and Ergonomic Challenges of Ventilating a Premature Infant During Delayed Cord Clamping. *Children* **2019**, *6*, 59. [CrossRef] [PubMed]
15. Bhatt, S.; Alison, B.J.; Wallace, E.M.; Crossley, K.J.; Gill, A.W.; Kluckow, M.; te Pas, A.B.; Morley, C.J.; Polglase, G.R.; Hooper, S.B. Delaying cord clamping until ventilation onset improves cardiovascular function at birth in preterm lambs. *J. Physiol.* **2013**, *591* Pt 8, 2113–2126. [CrossRef]
16. Ersdal, H.L.; Linde, J.; Mduma, E.; Auestad, B.; Perlman, J. Neonatal Outcome Following Cord Clamping After Onset of Spontaneous Respiration. *Pediatrics* **2014**, *134*, 265–272. [CrossRef] [PubMed]
17. Thomas, M.R.; Yoxall, C.W.; Weeks, A.D.; Duley, L. Providing newborn resuscitation at the mother's bedside: Assessing the safety, usability and acceptability of a mobile trolley. *BMC Pediatr.* **2014**, *14*, 135. [CrossRef] [PubMed]
18. Katheria, A.; Lee, H.C.; Knol, R.; Irvine, L.; Thomas, S. A review of different resuscitation platforms during delayed cord clamping. *J. Perinatol.* **2021**, 1–9. [CrossRef]
19. Knol, R.; Brouwer, E.; Klumper, F.J.C.M.; van den Akker, T.; DeKoninck, P.; Hutten, G.J.; Lopriore, E.; van Kaam, A.H.; Polglase, G.R.; Reiss, I.K.M.; et al. Effectiveness of Stabilization of Preterm Infants With Intact Umbilical Cord Using a Purpose-Built Resuscitation Table—Study Protocol for a Randomized Controlled Trial. *Front. Pediatr* **2019**, *7*, 134. [CrossRef] [PubMed]
20. Irvine, L.; Kowal, D.; Soraisham, A.; Cooper, S.; Stritzke, A.; Rabi, Y. Integrated Neonatal Support on Placental Circulation with Resuscitation (INSPiRe): A Feasibility Study. In Proceedings of the 10th American Pediatrics Healthcare & Pediatric Infectious Diseases Congress, Toronto, ON, Canada, 20–22 September 2017.
21. Katheria, A.C.; Sorkhi, S.R.; Hassen, K.; Faksh, A.; Ghorishi, Z.; Poeltler, D. Acceptability of Bedside Resuscitation with Intact Umbilical Cord to Clinicians and Patients' Families in the United States. *Front. Pediatr.* **2018**, *6*, 100. [CrossRef] [PubMed]

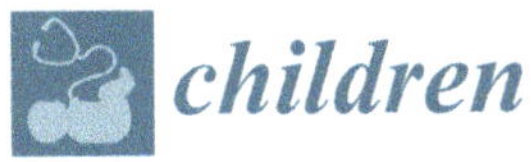

Article

Maintaining Normothermia in Preterm Babies during Stabilisation with an Intact Umbilical Cord

Alexander James Cleator, Emma Coombe, Vasiliki Alexopoulou, Laura Levingston, Kathryn Evans, Jonathan Christopher Hurst [iD] and Charles William Yoxall *[iD]

Liverpool Women's Hospital, Liverpool L8 7SS, UK; acleator@doctors.org.uk (A.J.C.); Emma.coombe2@lwh.nhs.uk (E.C.); v.alexopoulou@nhs.net (V.A.); laura.levingston@lwh.nhs.uk (L.L.); Kathryn.evans@lwh.nhs.uk (K.E.); Jonathan.hurst@lwh.nhs.uk (J.C.H.)
* Correspondence: bilyox@liverpool.ac.uk

Abstract: Background: We had experienced an increase in admission hypothermia rates during implementation of deferred cord clamping (DCC) in our unit. Our objective was to reduce the number of babies with a gestation below 32 weeks who are hypothermic on admission, whilst practising DCC and providing delivery room cuddles (DRC). Method: A 12 month quality improvement project set, in a large Neonatal Intensive Care Unit, from January 2020 to December 2020. Monthly rates of admission hypothermia (<36.5 °C) for all eligible babies, were tracked prospectively. Each hypothermic baby was reviewed as part of a series of Plan, Do, Study Act (PDSA) cycles, to understand potential reasons and to develop solutions. Implementation of these solutions included the dissemination of the learning through a variety of methods. The main outcome measure was the proportion of babies who were hypothermic (<36.5 °C) on admission compared to the previous 12 months. Results: 130 babies with a gestation below 32 weeks were admitted during the study period. 90 babies (69.2%) had DCC and 79 babies (60%) received DRC. Compared to the preceding 12 months, the rate of hypothermia decreased from 25/109 (22.3%) to 13/130 (10%) ($p = 0.017$). Only 1 baby (0.8%) was admitted with a temperature below 36 °C and 12 babies (9.2%) were admitted with a temperature between 36 °C and 36.4 °C. Continued monitoring during the 3 months after the end of the project showed that the improvements were sustained with 0 cases of hypothermia in 33 consecutive admissions. Conclusions: It is possible to achieve low rates of admission hypothermia in preterm babies whilst providing DCC and DRC. Using a quality improvement approach with PDSA cycles is an effective method of changing clinical practice to improve outcomes.

Keywords: hypothermia; umbilical cord; preterm; resuscitation

Citation: Cleator, A.J.; Coombe, E.; Alexopoulou, V.; Levingston, L.; Evans, K.; Hurst, J.C.; Yoxall, C.W. Maintaining Normothermia in Preterm Babies during Stabilisation with an Intact Umbilical Cord. *Children* **2022**, *9*, 75. https://doi.org/10.3390/children9010075

Academic Editors: Simone Pratesi, David Hutchon and Anup Katheria

Received: 13 December 2021
Accepted: 29 December 2021
Published: 5 January 2022

Publisher's Note: MDPI stays neutral with regard to jurisdictional claims in published maps and institutional affiliations.

1. Introduction

Preterm babies are particularly vulnerable to hypothermia after birth. Hypothermia is an independent risk factor for death [1,2] and a risk factor for the development of respiratory distress syndrome, intraventricular haemorrhage, late onset sepsis and severe neurodevelopmental impairment [3,4].

The benefits of Deferred Cord Clamping (DCC) at preterm birth are well documented, including a reduction in hospital mortality [5].

Across the UK, in 2018 only 5.2% of babies with a gestation below 32 weeks had a documented period of DCC lasting for 60 s or more (Data from Badger System, Clevermed, UK. Personal communication, CEO, Clevermed, Edinburgh, UK). Our unit has been an early adopter of DCC. We recruited babies into studies to evaluate the practicability of using the Lifestart trolley to facilitate DCC in 2012 and 2013 [6] and enrolled babies into a randomised controlled trial of DCC from 2013 to 2015 [7]. There was some practise of DCC subsequently, but following the publication of the trial evidence showing clear benefit, we undertook a quality improvement project and increased the rate of DCC for at least 120 s to 92% of eligible babies in 2018 and 2019 [8]. During that period of implementation, we noted an increase in the rate of admission hypothermia (<36.5 °C) to 20% from a previous stable baseline rate of 12% (Figure 1).

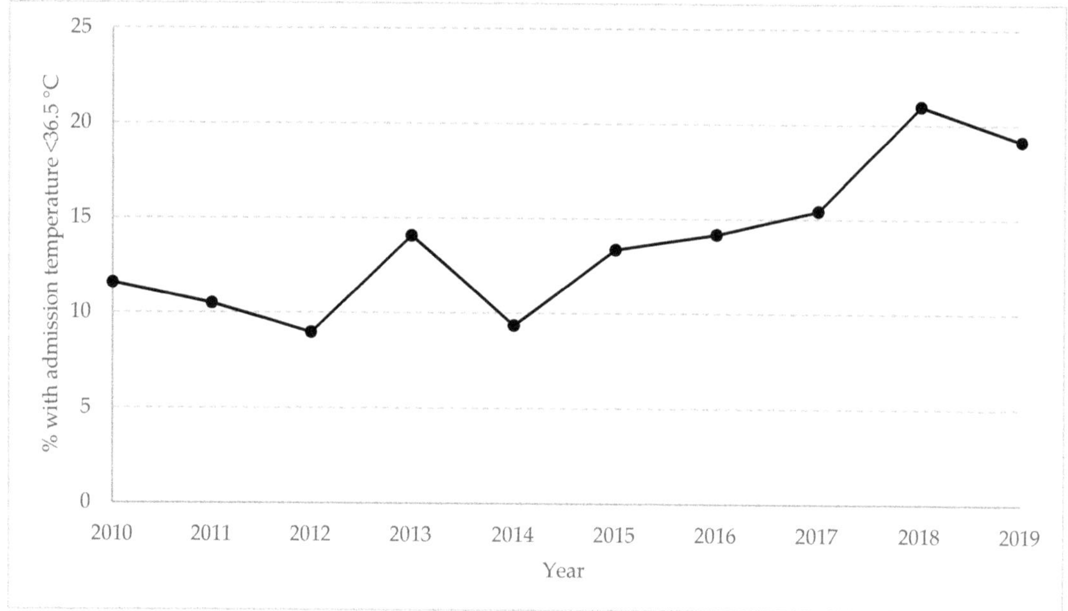

Figure 1. Proportion of babies born before 32 weeks gestation with an admission temperature below 36.5 °C across time during the introduction of DCC on our unit.

In addition to promoting DCC, we have also recently started providing delivery room cuddles (DRC) following stabilisation of the baby. Once the baby is stable, a brief period of physical contact with the parents takes place before transfer to the neonatal unit. This can be achieved whilst the baby is receiving respiratory support. Two recent randomised controlled trials have shown reductions in both post-partum depression and mother-infant bonding problems following DRC [9,10], although one trial [10] found lower temperatures one hour after birth in their DRC group.

The UK National Neonatal Audit Project (NNAP) standard relating to admission temperature for preterm babies states that 90% of babies born <32 weeks should have a temperature between 36.5 °C and 37.5 °C when first admitted to the Neonatal Intensive care Unit (NICU), i.e., requires avoidance of hyperthermia as well as hypothermia.

The aim of this project was to reduce the number of preterm babies who are hypothermic (temperature < 36.5 °C) on admission to our neonatal unit, whilst promoting and practising DCC and DRC. In view of the NNAP standard, rates of admission hyperthermia were also measured.

2. Materials and Methods

We aimed to provide stabilisation at birth with at least 2 min of DCC in all babies born before 32 weeks gestation. The period of 2 min was the same as that used in the Cord Pilot trial (7). DCC is provided in our unit using the LifeStart trolley (Inspirations Healthcare, Crawley, UK) in the delivery room. This is a resuscitation platform that facilitates stabilisation of the preterm baby whilst the umbilical cord remains intact. This device has been described in detail in recent literature [6,11].

In addition, we aimed to provide DRC for all babies once stabilised, prior to moving the baby to the NICU. Once a baby was stable, with acceptable heart rate, oxygen saturation and appropriate thermal care in place, the baby was passed to the mother for a period of physical contact lasting up to 5 min. This was not skin-to-skin care. The baby continued to receive care wrapped in a plastic bag and in contact with a self heating gel mattress (Transwarmer (Drager Medical, Hemel Hempstead, UK)) if appropriate, they were also wrapped in warmed towels and a hat was in place. This period of contact was achieved for babies who were receiving respiratory support using continuous airway pressure (CPAP) (Figure 2) and in babies who were ventilated following tracheal intubation. In some families, the period of cuddling was shared with the father and following delivery by caesarean section under general anaesthetic, the cuddle was offered to the father alone if he was present.

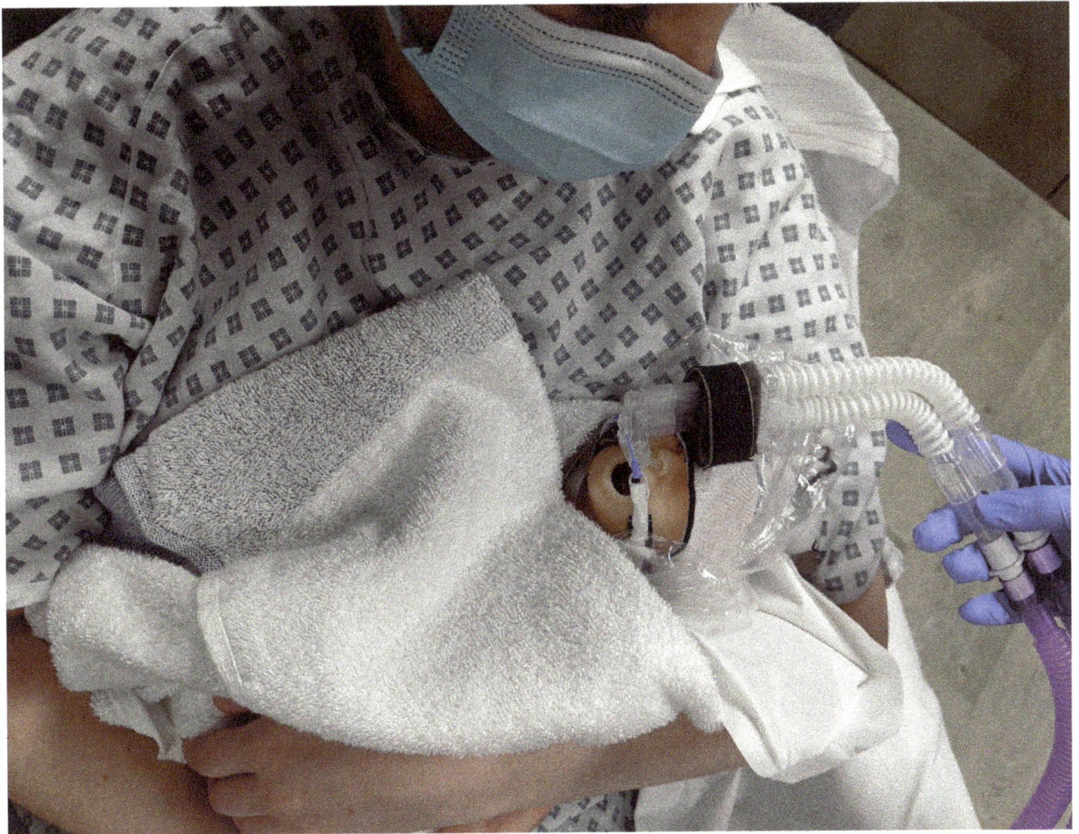

Figure 2. Simulation of a preterm baby receiving Delivery Room Cuddles whilst receiving respiratory support with nasal CPAP.

We completed a 12-month quality improvement programme (QIP) from January 2020 to December 2020. Data were collected manually and from the electronic patient record (Badgernet full EPR, Clevermed, Edinburgh, UK) following the delivery of all babies born at less than 32 weeks' gestation. For the purposes of this project, we used the World Health Organisation definitions [2] to classify babies into 5 temperature groups; severely hypothermic (<32 °C), moderately hypothermic (32–35.9 °C), cold stress (36–36.4 °C), normothermic (36.5–37.5 °C) or hyperthermic (>37.5 °C). Axillary temperature was measured in all babies at all times using an electronic thermometer (Welsh Allyn Suretemp Plus, Welsh Allyn, Buckinghamshire UK).

A multidisciplinary team (MDT) was assembled consisting of neonatal consultants, trainees, nurse practitioners and neonatal nurses. The proportion of babies in each temperature group was measured monthly. A detailed review was conducted for each baby who had an admission temperature below 36.5 °C. The MDT met monthly and reviewed all data including the birth location, presentation at birth and mode of delivery as well as the weight and gestation of all babies who were hypothermic or hyperthermic to try to identify common associations with these outcomes. Most importantly, interviews were conducted with the staff responsible for or involved in providing the baby's care during stabilisation and transfer to gain their views on what they thought they could do differently in the future similar circumstances to prevent this outcome. Strategies to implement better thermoregulation practice were formulated by the MDT based on these data.

A series of Plan, Do, Study, Act (PDSA) cycles were performed using a standard methodology [12]. PDSA cycles are an iterative method of quality improvement that are used sequentially to change practice in order to improve outcomes. The basic structure of a PDSA cycle is:

Plan—to define what clinical practice should be to achieve the best outcome based on what we know about the subject. Decide what data are required to study the outcome (performance metric) and to establish a system of data collection.

Do—to implement best practice and collect the data prospectively.

Study—to review the data and assess performance against the metric and understand what the causes of underperformance are.

Act—to make recommendations about changes in practice to improve performance and plan the next cycle.

Not all of the PDSA cycles we undertook were synchronous. Once the project was commenced (the initial P and D phases), there was a monthly review of data (S) and new actions were taken if the MDT were able to make a new recommendation (A). Each intervention was then planned (P) and implemented (D). During some meetings new cycles could be started before a previous cycle had completed (e.g., recommendations about managing twins on the Lifestart trolley were made in June, but we needed several sets of twins to be born in order to assess the effectiveness of this, in the meantime we implemented other changes in practice). Similarly, new actions were not implemented at every monthly meeting as no new changes in practice could be recommended based on the data available at that time.

Communication of changes in practice to the clinical staff required to implement them is a key part of the "Do" phase of the PDSA cycle. In this study each new strategy was communicated to the staff on the unit through a variety of methods:

- The performance data generated each month were displayed graphically in a bi-monthly newsletter which also summarised new practice changes implemented.
- 'Top tips' posters communicating key changes in practice were produced.
- A range of methods of information dissemination were used to reach staff who accessed information in different ways. The newsletters and 'Top tips' posters were displayed across the neonatal unit, appeared on the unit's social media pages and were emailed to all medical and nursing staff.
- The unit's education team incorporated all new changes into staff induction and annual update teaching.
- We reinforced important messages or changes in practice using the unit's system of "lesson of the week" announcements made at each shift handover.
- Written unit policies were amended to include new changes in practice as appropriate.

Some interventions also required liaison with our colleagues in other departments such as maternity and medical engineering.

The project was performed in a large women's hospital in the UK which houses a tertiary NICU. Comparisons were made with the rates of hypothermia seen on our unit in the preceding 12 months. The statistical significance of any differences were tested using Chi-squared with Yates correction. Performance data were also collected for a 3 month period following the end of the intervention period to assess the impact of interventions made in the latter part of the period. The project was approved by the Institutional Clinical Effectiveness Senate (approval date 15 November 2019, approval number QIP 0058).

3. Results

130 babies less than 32 weeks' gestation were admitted to the unit between January 2020 and December 2020. The median (range) gestation was 29 (22 to 31) completed weeks. The median (range) Birth Weight was 1225 (510 to 2810) grams.

In total 90 babies (69.2%) received DCC with 69 (53%) receiving a least 2 min of DCC and 21 (16.1%) receiving between 1 and 2 min of DCC. During this period we also successfully implemented Delivery Room Cuddles (DRC) with 79 (60%) of the babies documented to have received this.

A number of thermoregulation strategies were implemented during the project during the PDSA cycles:

- Based on the performance data from 2019, the MDT made some immediate changes to practice at the start of the QIP intervention period (January 2020). These included:
  - Hats for all preterm babies—We noticed that some babies who were not receiving respiratory support were not having a hat applied after birth. Subsequent routine practice included putting a hat on all babies as soon as possible.
  - An increase in the use of plastic bags to maintain normothermia from our previous gestation threshold of 30 weeks to 32 weeks.
  - An increase in the use of self heating gel mattresses to maintain normothermia from our previous gestation threshold of 28 weeks to 30 weeks.
- March 2020: Temperature checks—on the basis of the data, we decided to measure 3 temperatures following delivery. The first was taken as soon as practically possible after birth, the second after DRC and the third on arrival to the unit. This allowed us to understand at what point during the stabilisation and transfer period the babies were moving out of range and to target our thermoregulation interventions.
- May 2020: The importance of activating the self heating gel mattress well in advance of the birth was recommended as there is a time delay before the peak temperature is reached.
- June 2020: Introduction of the Neohelp bag (Vygon, Swindon, UK)—This is a double walled plastic bag with a hood and a Velcro opening at the front which allows the cord to remain intact whilst keeping the baby covered. This device was found to be effective and so was introduced into our regular practice for all babies born before 32 weeks.
- June 2020: Lifestart trolley at multiple births—we reviewed the optimal way to use a single Lifestart trolley at a multiple preterm birth. Detailed instructions for best practice was disseminated using a "Top Tips" poster (Figure 3).
- June 2020: (following a period of evaluation of practicability in May): Use of a non-interruptible power supply for the overhead heater during transfer to the neonatal unit. On our unit, babies are transferred from the labour ward to the neonatal unit using a Panda resuscitation platform (GE Healthcare, Buckinghamshire, UK). We found that some babies were becoming cold during transfer. The Panda can be attached to a non-interruptible power supply using a device called 'The Shuttle' (GE Healthcare, Buckinghamshire, UK). This allowed the overhead heater to remain on during transfer to the neonatal unit.

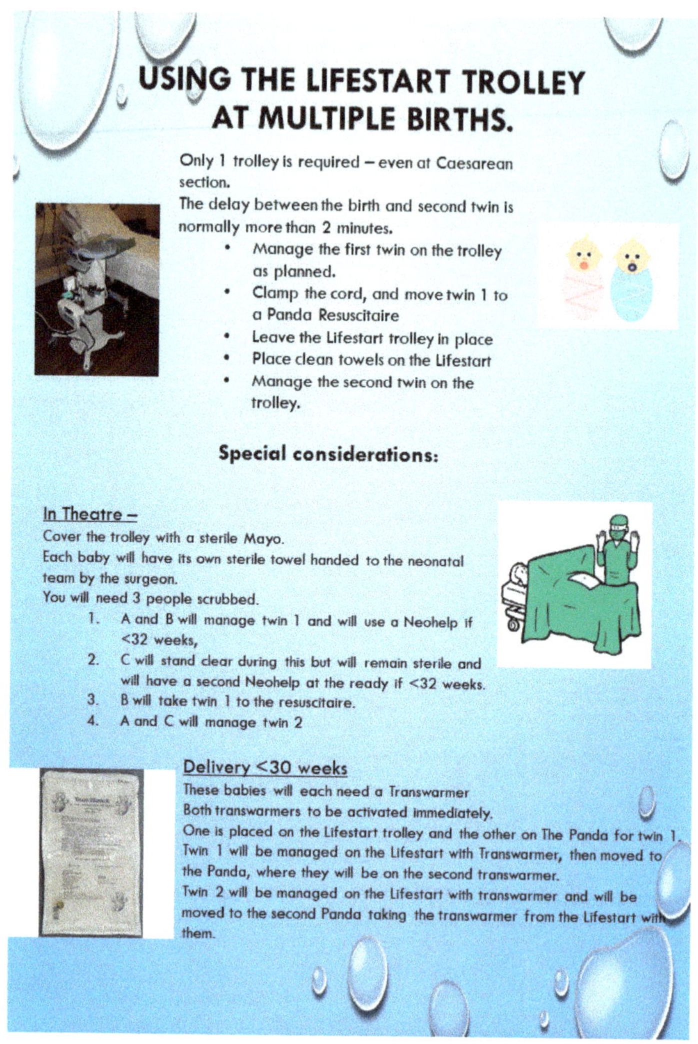

Figure 3. An example of a "Top Tips" poster used to communicate best practice to staff.

- October 2020: For babies born in theatre, we found that the transwarmer underneath the sterile drape was often left behind when transferring the baby to the resuscitation platform. Subsequently we used two transwarmers for delivery in theatre; one was placed underneath the sterile drape that covers the LifeStart whilst the baby was receiving care with an intact umbilical cord and one was placed on the Panda resuscitation platform used for further stabilisation and transfer to the neonatal unit.
- November 2020: Breech deliveries—the data showed that several babies born by vaginal breech delivery were hypothermic despite the above interventions. Following a discussion with the obstetric team, we agreed to cover the body of babies born as breech deliveries with the Neohelp bag whilst waiting for the head to be delivered.
- November 2020: Turning down the overhead heater—in babies who had a post DRC temperature of >37.5 °C, the overhead heater was reduced to 50% power prior to leaving for the neonatal unit.

The proportion of babies in each of the temperature groups during each month of the project is shown in Figure 4. The proportion of babies in each month that had hypothermia is shown in Figure 5. Assessing the individual impact of each of the new strategies that we introduced is difficult because of the time lag between each intervention and outcome and the non-synchronous nature of the PDSA cycles. The cumulative impact of the project is demonstrated in these charts which show a reduction in the rate of hypothermia during the latter part of the QIP period and into the following 3 months.

We have compared temperature outcomes from the babies admitted during the QIP intervention period with the 109 babies less than 32 weeks' gestation born between January 2019 and December 2019. The lower number in the 2019 cohort was a consequence of normal variation in unit activity. The distribution of babies by temperature group between the two cohorts is shown in Figure 6.

During the QIP intervention period there were no cases of severe hypothermia (<32 °C), only 1 baby (0.77%) was admitted with moderate hypothermia (32–35.9 °C) and 12 babies (9.2%) were admitted with cold stress (36–36.4 °C). When compared to the 2019 cohort, there has been a significant reduction in babies admitted with a temperature below 36.5 °C from 22.3% to 10% ($p = 0.006$). This improvement was maintained after the intervention period. The rate of hypothermia in the last 6 months of data collection (last 3 months of the QIP intervention period plus the following 3 months) was 4/73 babies (5.5%). There were no hypothermic babies in the first 3 months after the QIP intervention period.

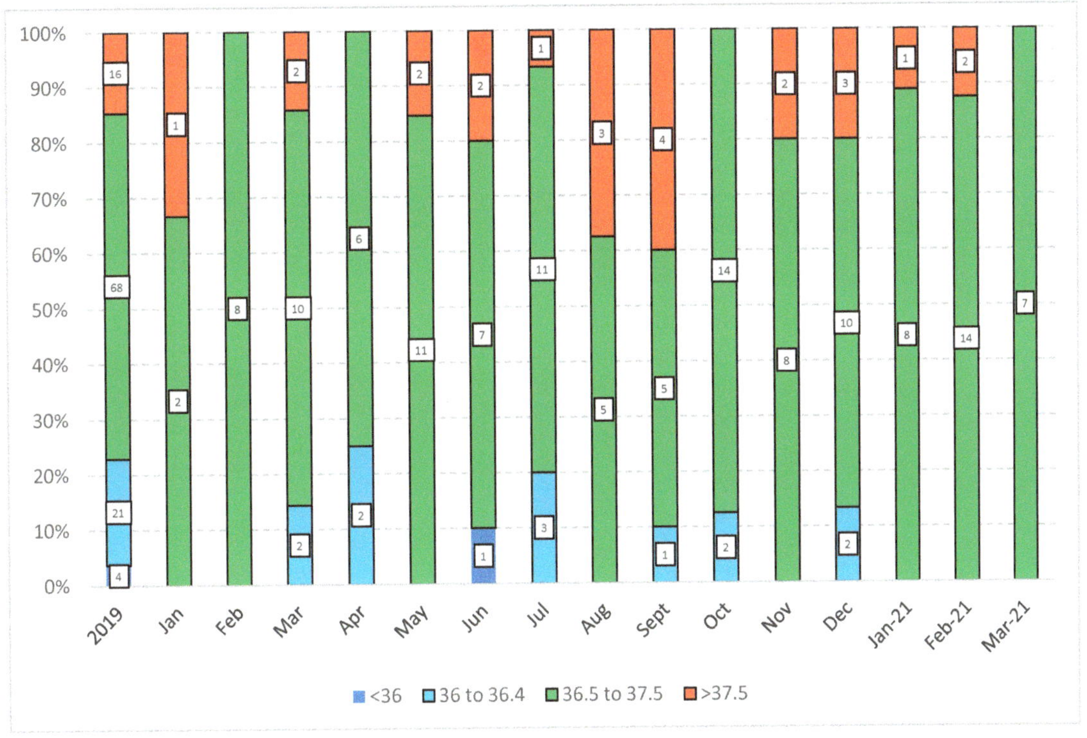

Figure 4. The proportion of babies admitted in each temperature category during 2019, each month of the QIP intervention period and during the 3 month period after the QIP intervention period. Numbers on the bars are absolute numbers in each category in each month.

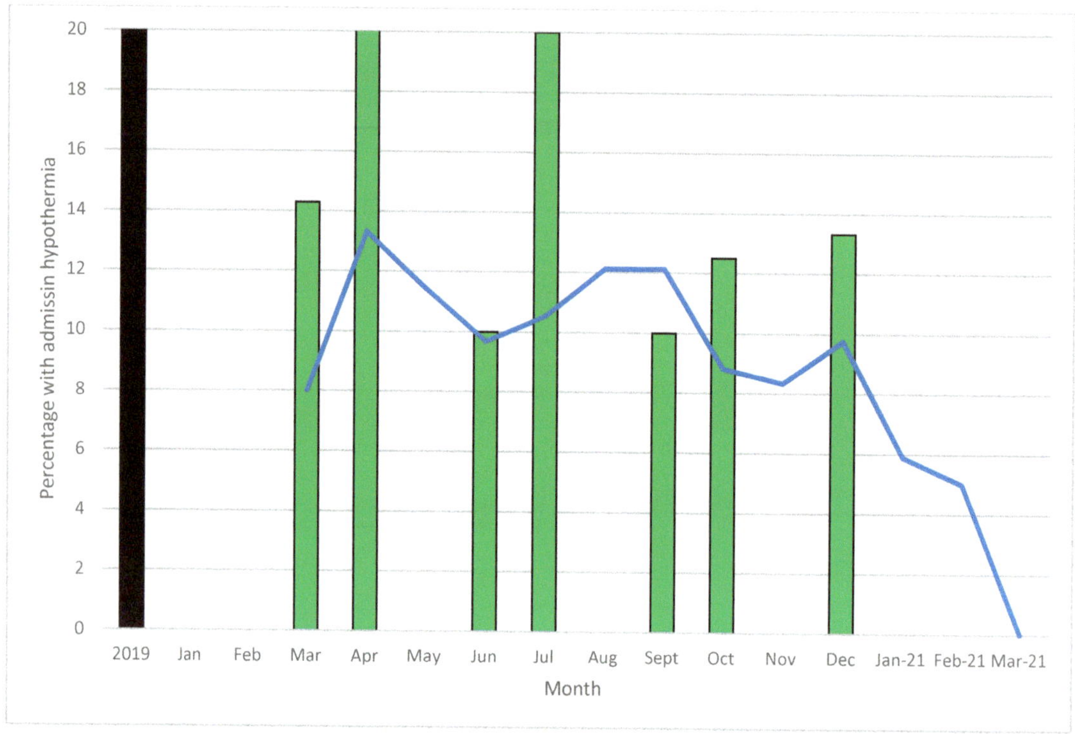

Figure 5. The percentage of babies with admission hypothermia in 2019 (black bar), during each month of the QIP intervention period (green bars) and during the 3 month period after the QIP intervention period (there were no hypothermic babies during this period). The blue line represents a 3 month rolling average.

There was a slight increase in the rate of admission hyperthermia from 14.7% (20/109) in 2019 to 15.4% (20/130) in 2020, although this increase was not statistically significant ($p = 0.88$). During the 3 months after the end of the QIP intervention period 3/32 (9.4%) of babies were hyperthermic.

We were interested to understand whether the hyperthermia was due to iatrogenic warming, or due to the prevention of heat loss in already pyrexial babies. We had introduced a policy of making multiple temperature measurements at specific times during the stabilisation and transfer period during the study as described above. There were 67 babies who had paired temperature measurements on the labour ward and on admission to the neonatal unit. 55 of these were normothermic on admission and 12 were hyperthermic. Babies who were hyperthermic on admission had higher temperatures measured during their stabilisation on labour ward (Figure 7). The median (range) temperature on labour ward of the babies who were hyperthermic on admission was 37.5 °C (36.9 °C to 38.7 °C), compared to 36.9 °C (36.1 °C to 38.2 °C) in the babies who were normothermic on admission ($p = 0.0004$). All but one of the babies who were hyperthermic on admission to the neonatal unit had a temperature on labour ward above 37 °C.

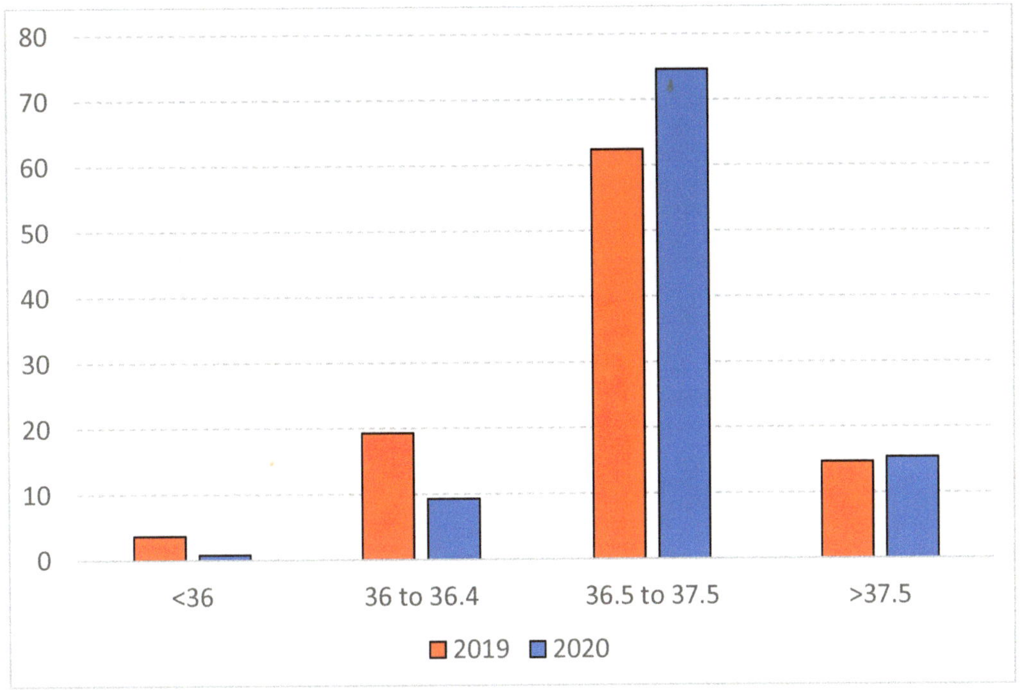

Figure 6. The distribution of babies between the different temperature categories in the 2019 cohort and the 2020 cohort.

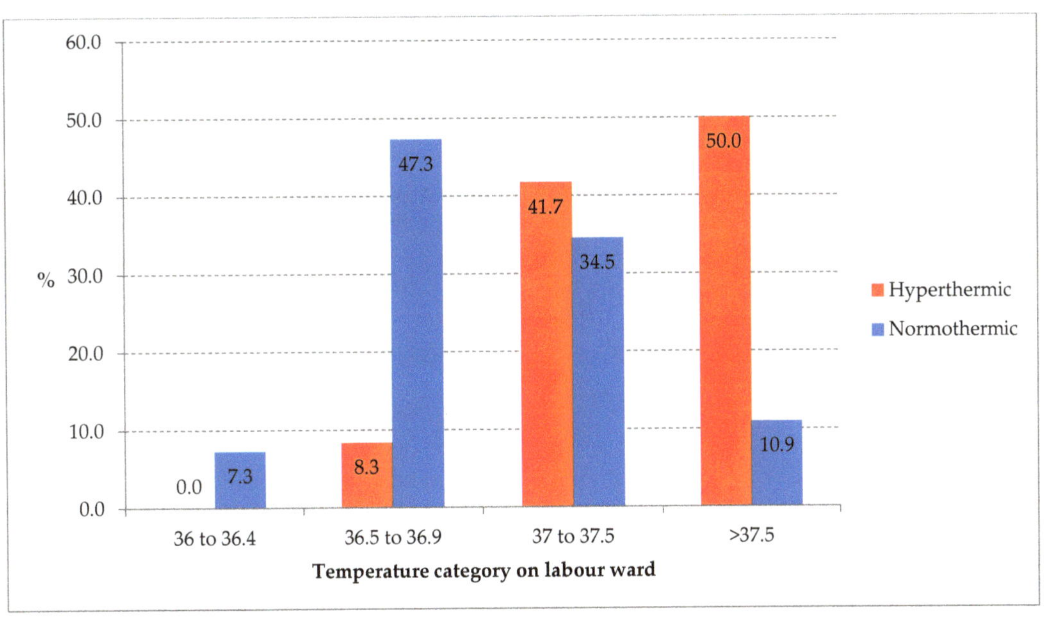

Figure 7. Temperature category at birth for babies who were normothermic on the labour ward (blue bars) and babies who were hyperthermic on the labour ward (red bars).

4. Discussion

Admission hypothermia is preventable by improved care, both in the delivery room and during the transfer to the neonatal unit. Our results have demonstrated that it is possible to almost eradicate significant admission hypothermia in a busy NICU. This is achievable whilst still practising DCC and DRC, both of which are beneficial in the immediate care of the newly born preterm baby.

The solutions that we have developed in our QIP may not be the best solutions in another environment and we recommend that other units adopt a similar approach to develop their own best solution. Our solution may provide a useful starting point however and we have included a "Step by Step guide" (Figure 8) which illustrates our learning during this project.

Ambient temperature was not recorded systematically during our project, so we are unable to comment on its role in hypothermia in our own population. Published standards state that a temperature of 23 °C to 25 °C should be achieved for the delivery room [13].

A systematic review of trials of deferred cord clamping found little evidence of an impact on admission temperature [5] so we did not expect to see the increase in admission hypothermia that we experienced when we implemented DCC into our practice. Further examination of the published admission temperature data from 7 trials in the systematic review however shows that, although there was little or no impact of DCC on admission temperature, the rate of hypothermia in both intervention and control groups was high. These data are summarised in Table 1. Data are reported as mean (SD) in each trial and the reported mean is below 36.7 in 5 of the 7 trials, with wide standard deviations, demonstrating that a significant proportion of the participants in both the intervention group and the control groups of these trials, were hypothermic on admission. The mean (SD) temperature on admission in our cohort was 37 (0.53) °C. Even in one of the trials reporting mean admission temperatures of above 36.5 °C [7], there were still 11.6% of babies with an admission temperature below 36 °C. Taken together, these observations suggest that in clinical areas where there are already moderate rates of admission hypothermia, the introduction of DCC makes little difference to these rates. Our experience, in a unit with a low rate of hypothermia, is that the introduction of DCC was associated with an increase in hypothermia.

Table 1. Published admission temperature data from randomized controlled trials of deferred cord clamping at preterm birth.

| Study | Subjects | Group Temperature Mean (SD) °C | | Comment |
		Control	Intervention	
Mercer [14]	32	36.3 (17.2)	36.3 (17.2)	Minimum temperatures reported were 35.2 °C in Control group and 34.7 °C in the intervention group
Mercer [15]	72	36 (0.8)	36.2 (6)	Minimum temperature reported were 33.8 °C in the control group and 34.4 °C in the intervention group
Backes [16]	40	35.7 (16.8)	36.3 (16.8)	
Dipak [17]	53	34 (0.7)	33.9 (0.8)	
Tarnow Mordi [18]	1248	36.4 (0.9)	36.3 (0.8)	
Duley [7]	266	36.9 (0.6)	36.7 (0.6)	31 (11.6%) trial subjects had admission temp <36 °C
Yunis [19]	60	36.8 (0.4)	36.7 (0.5)	

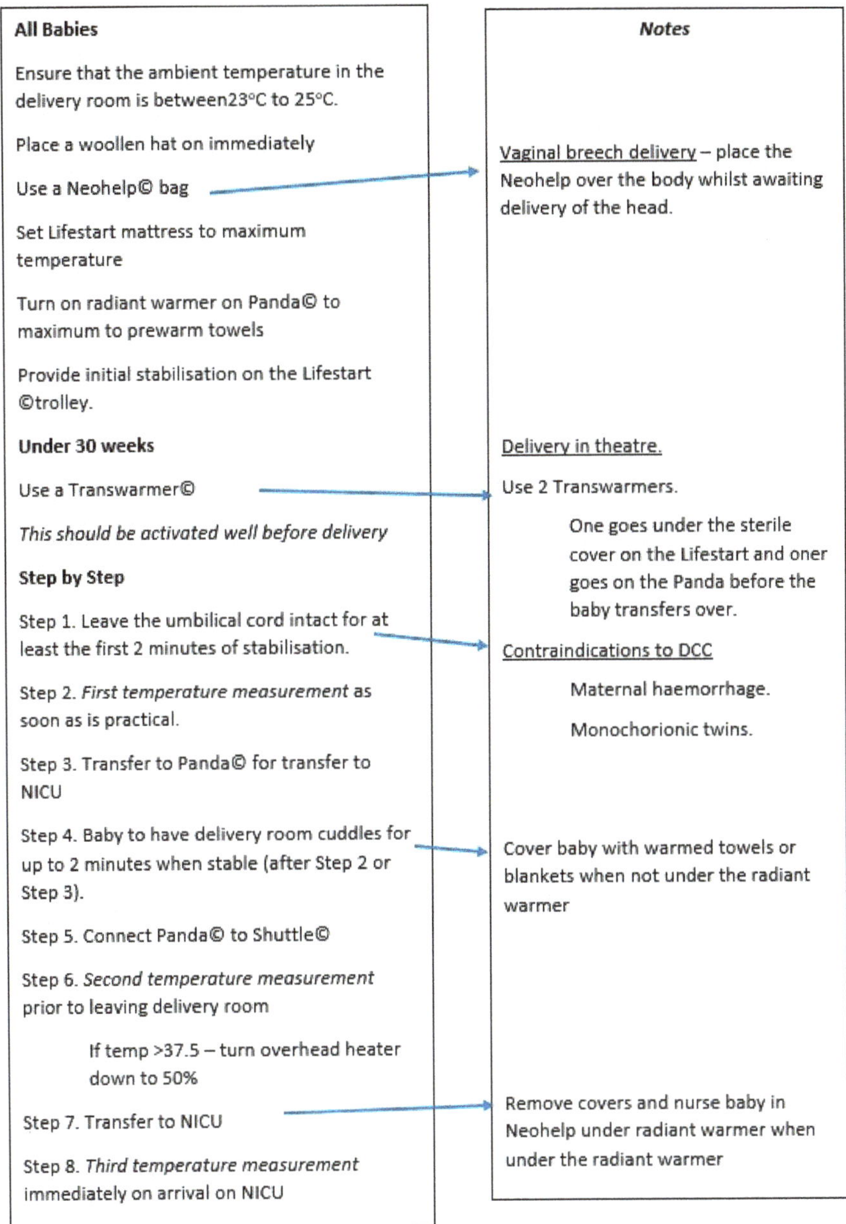

Figure 8. A Step by Step Guide to maintaining normothermia during preterm stabilisation with an intact umbilical cord, summarising all of our learning during this project.

Despite the significant reductions in hypothermia we achieved, we failed to achieve the NNAP standard of 90% of babies in the normothermic range during the QIP intervention period, although that was achieved in one of the subsequent 3 months (Figure 9). During the QIP intervention period, the commonest cause of failing to meet the NNAP standard was hyperthermia (n = 20) rather than hypothermia (n = 13). Our exploration of the data, presented above, shows that much, if not all, of the admission hyperthermia we saw was a consequence of prevention of heat loss in already pyrexial babies rather than iatrogenic warming.

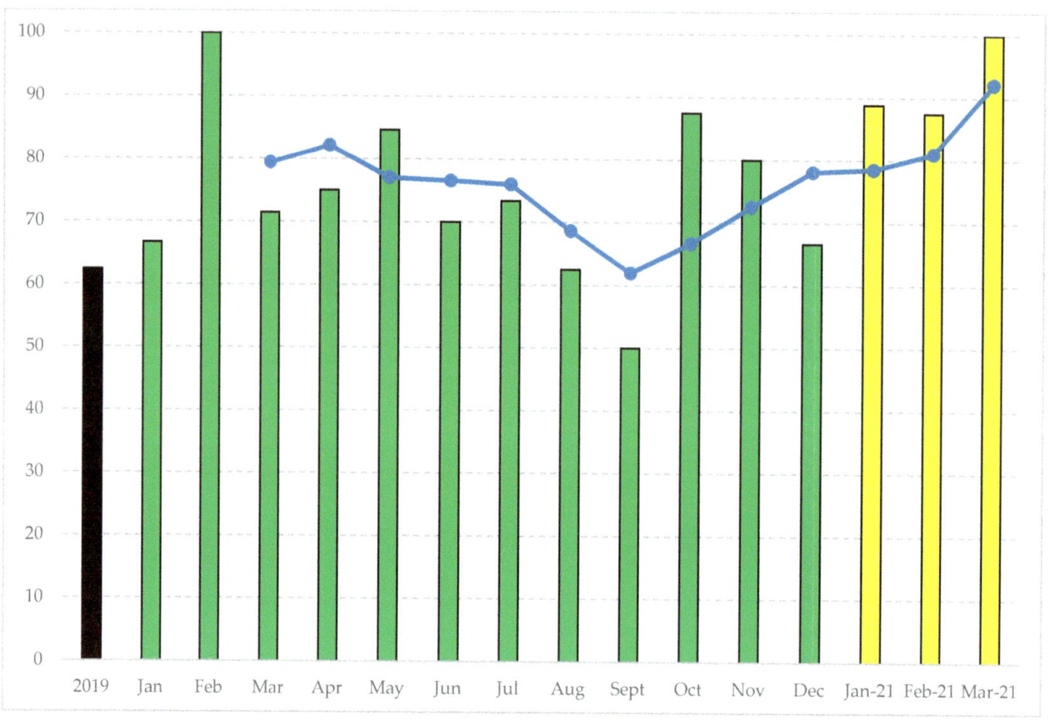

Figure 9. Compliance with the NNAP standard by month during 2019 (black bar), each month during the QIP intervention period (green bars) and each of the 3 months immediately after the QIP intervention period (yellow bars). The blue line represents a 3 month rolling average.

Although the evidence for a causal relationship between hypothermia and adverse outcome at preterm birth is well established and accepted, the evidence relating to hyperthermia is not compelling. In fact, there is little published evidence in relation to this matter. Lyu et al. found an increased rate of a composite adverse outcome (severe neurological injury, severe retinopathy of prematurity, necrotising enterocolitis, bronchopulmonary dysplasia, and nosocomial infection) in babies with an admission temperature above 38 °C [20]. Sharma et al. also reported an increase in a composite adverse outcome (mortality or major morbidity) in babies with admission temperature >37.5 °C [21]. The Clinical Risk Indicator for Babies II score (CRIB II) [22] assigns an increased score (increased risk of mortality) to babies with an admission temperature >37.5 °C. We assume that this is because the dataset on which the score was developed found an increased risk of death in those babies, although this is not explicitly stated in the paper describing the development of the score. Although these studies provide some evidence of an association between hyperthermia on admission and adverse outcome in preterm babies, none of the published studies has established a causal link and it is possible that this association is due a shared aetiology with chorioamnionitis, which also has a strong association with preterm brain injury [23,24]. The 2020 International Liaison Committee on Resuscitation recommendations for neonatal life support include a weak recommendation, based on low certainty evidence, that hyperthermia (greater than 38 °C) should be avoided due to the potential associated risks [13]. On this basis we believe that a small increase in hyperthermia is probably an acceptable consequence of a reduction in hypothermia. Nonetheless, we still strive to avoid hyperthermia by switching off the power supply to the overhead heather during transfer of babies with a temperature following DRC above 37 °C as described above.

5. Conclusions

This project highlights the importance of the perinatal MDT for driving change in a large complex organisation. Collaboration and clear communication with our obstetric, midwifery, medical engineering and estate staff colleagues were vital to facilitating the success of this project. We have used this approach previously to successfully drive change in our unit [8,25]. The team approach (rather than a top-down approach) promotes ownership of the project, generates enthusiasm and helps create a genuine desire for success.

Author Contributions: Conceptualization, C.W.Y.; methodology, C.W.Y.; investigation, A.J.C., E.C., V.A., L.L., K.E., J.C.H., C.W.Y.; writing—original draft preparation, A.J.C.; writing—review and editing, C.W.Y.; supervision, C.W.Y.; project administration, C.W.Y.; funding acquisition, C.W.Y. All authors have read and agreed to the published version of the manuscript.

Funding: This study received no external funding.

Institutional Review Board Statement: The project was approved by the Institutional Clinical Effectiveness Senate at Liverpool Women's Hospital (approval number QIP 0058).

Informed Consent Statement: Patient consent was waived as this study was performed using existing clinical data with no allocation of individuals to any intervention.

Data Availability Statement: The data presented in this study are available in the text and tables of this manuscript.

Acknowledgments: Publication costs of this study were supported by Inspiration Healthcare. Thanks to Emily Hoyle for providing the photograph in Figure 1, along with K.E.

Conflicts of Interest: C.W.Y. arranged for publication costs of this study to be funded by Inspiration Healthcare. The funders had no role in the design of the study; in the collection, analyses, or interpretation of data; in the writing of the manuscript, or in the decision to publish the results. There are no other conflict.

References

1. Wilson, E.; Maier, R.F.; Norman, M.; Misselwitz, B.; Howell, E.A.; Zeitlin, J.; Bonamy, A.K.; Van Reempts, P.; Martens, E.; Martens, G.; et al. Admission hypothermia in very preterm infants and neonatal mortality and morbidity. *J. Pediatr.* **2016**, *175*, 61–67. [CrossRef]
2. World Health Organization, Department of Reproductive Health Research. *Thermal Protection of the Newborn: A Practical Guide*; Division of Reproductive Health (Technical Support), World Health Organization: Geneva, Switzerland, 1997; p. 56.
3. Ting, J.Y.; Synnes, A.R.; Lee, S.K.; Shah, P.S.; Canadian Neonatal Network and Canadian Neonatal Follow-Up Network. Association of admission temperature and death or adverse neurodevelopmental outcomes in extremely low-gestational age neonates. *J. Perinatol.* **2018**, *38*, 844–849. [CrossRef]
4. Yu, Y.H.; Wang, L.; Huang, L.; Wang, L.L.; Huang, X.Y.; Fan, X.F.; Ding, Y.J.; Zhang, C.Y.; Liu, Q.; Sun, A.R.; et al. Association between admission hypothermia and outcomes in very low birth weight infants in China: A multicentre prospective study. *BMC Pediatr.* **2020**, *20*, 321. [CrossRef]
5. Fogarty, M.; Osborn, D.A.; Askie, L.; Seidler, A.L.; Hunter, K.; Lui, K.; Simes, J.; Tarnow-Mordi, W. Delayed vs early umbilical cord clamping for preterm infants: A systematic review and meta-analysis. *Am. J. ObstetGynecol.* **2018**, *218*, 118. [CrossRef] [PubMed]
6. Thomas, M.R.; Yoxall, C.W.; Weeks, A.D.; Duley, L. Providing newborn resuscitation at the mother's bedside: Assessing the safety, usability and acceptability of a mobile trolley. *BMC Pediatr.* **2014**, *14*, 135. [CrossRef] [PubMed]
7. Duley, L.; Dorling, J.; Pushpa-Rajah, A.; Oddie, S.J.; Yoxall, C.W.; Schoonakker, B.; Bradshaw, L.; Mitchell, E.J.; Fawke, J.A. Randomised trial of cord clamping and initial stabilisation at very preterm birth. *Arch. Dis. Child. Fetal Neonatal Ed.* **2018**, *103*, F6–F14. [CrossRef] [PubMed]

8. Hoyle, E.S.; Hirani, S.; Ogden, S.; Deeming, J.; Yoxall, C.W. Quality improvement programme to increase the rate of deferred cord clamping at preterm birth using the Lifestart trolley. *Arch. Dis. Child. Fetal Neonatal Ed.* **2020**, *105*, 652–655. [CrossRef]
9. Mehler, K.; Hucklenbruch-Rother, E.; Trautmann-Villalba, P.; Becker, I.; Roth, B.; Kribs, A. Delivery room skin-to-skin contact for preterm infants-A randomized clinical trial. *Acta Paediatr.* **2020**, *109*, 518–526. [CrossRef]
10. Linnér, A.; Klemming, S.; Sundberg, B.; Lilliesköld, S.; Westrup, B.; Jonas, W.; Skiöld, B. Immediate skin-to-skin contact is feasible for very preterm infants but thermal control remains a challenge. *Acta Paediatr.* **2020**, *109*, 697–704. [CrossRef]
11. Weeks, A.D.; Watt, P.; Yoxall, C.W.; Gallagher, A.; Burleigh, A.; Bewley, S.; Heuchan, A.M.; Duley, L. Innovation in immediate neonatal care: Development of the Bedside Assessment, Stabilisation and Initial Cardiorespiratory Support (BASICS) trolley. *BMJ Innov.* **2015**, *1*, 53–58. [CrossRef] [PubMed]
12. Plan, Do, Study, Act (PDSA) Cycles and the Model for Improvement. Online Library of Quality, Service Improvement and Redesign Tools. NHS England and NHS Improvement. Available online: https://www.england.nhs.uk/wp-content/uploads/2021/03/qsir-plan-do-study-act.pdf (accessed on 11 December 2012).
13. Wyckoff, M.H.; Wyllie, J.; Aziz, K.; de Almeida, M.F.; Fabres, J.; Fawke, J.; Guinsburg, R.; Hosono, S.; Isayama, T.; Kapadia, V.S.; et al. Neonatal Life Support 2020 International Consensus on Cardiopulmonary Resuscitation and Emergency Cardiovascular Care Science With Treatment Recommendations. *Resuscitation* **2020**, *156*, A156–A187. [CrossRef]
14. Mercer, J.S.; McGrath, M.M.; Hensman, A.; Silver, H.; Oh, W. Immediate and delayed cord clamping in infants born between 24 and 32 weeks: A pilot randomized controlled trial. *J. Perinatol.* **2003**, *23*, 466–472. [CrossRef]
15. Mercer, J.S.; Vohr, B.R.; McGrath, M.M.; Padbury, J.F.; Wallach, M.; Oh, W. Delayed cord clamping in very preterm infants reduces the incidence of intraventricular hemorrhage and late-onset sepsis: A randomized, controlled trial. *Pediatrics* **2006**, *117*, 1235–1242. [CrossRef]
16. Backes, C.H.; Huang, H.; Iams, J.D.; Bauer, J.A.; Giannone, P.J. Timing of umbilical cord clamping among infants born at 22 through 27 weeks' gestation. *J. Perinatol.* **2016**, *36*, 35–40. [CrossRef] [PubMed]
17. Dipak, N.K.; Nanavat, R.N.; Kabra, N.K.; Srinivasan, A.; Ananthan, A. Effect of Delayed Cord Clamping on Hematocrit, and Thermal and Hemodynamic Stability in Preterm Neonates: A Randomized Controlled Trial. *Indian Pediatr.* **2017**, *54*, 112–115. [CrossRef]
18. Tarnow-Mordi, W.; Morris, J.; Kirby, A.; Robledo, K.; Askie, L.; Brown, R.; Evans, N.; Finlayson, S.; Fogarty, M.; Gebski, V.; et al. Delayed versus Immediate Cord Clamping in Preterm Infants. *N. Engl. J. Med.* **2017**, *377*, 2445–2455. [CrossRef]
19. Yunis, M.; Nour, I.; Gibreel, A.; Darwish, M.; Sarhan, M.; Shouman, B.; Nasef, N. Effect of delayed cord clamping on stem cell transfusion and hematological parameters in preterm infants with placental insufficiency: A pilot randomized trial. *Eur. J. Pediatr.* **2021**, *180*, 157–166. [CrossRef]
20. Lyu, Y.; Shah, P.S.; Xiang, Y.Y.; Warre, R.; Piedboeuf, B.; Deshpandey, A.; Dunn, M.; Lee, S.K.; Canadian Neonatal Network. Association between admission temperature and mortality and major morbidity in preterm infants born at fewer than 33 weeks' gestation. *JAMA Pediatr.* **2015**, *169*, e150277. [CrossRef] [PubMed]
21. Sharma, D.; Murki, S.; Pratap, T.; Deshbotla, S.K.; Vardhelli, V.; Pawale, D.; Kulkarni, D.; Arun, S.; Bashir, T.; Anne, R.P. Association between admission temperature and mortality and major morbidity in very low birth weight neonates—Single center prospective observational study. *J. Matern. Fetal Neonatal. Med.* **2020**, *24*, 1–9. [CrossRef]
22. Parry, G.; Tucker, J.; Tarnow-Mordi, W.; UK Neonatal Staffing Study Collaborative Group. CRIB II: An update of the clinical risk index for babies score. *Lancet* **2003**, *361*, 1789–1791. [CrossRef]
23. Strunk, T.; Inder, T.; Wang, X.; Burgner, D.; Mallard, C.; Levy, O. Infection-induced inflammation and cerebral injury in preterm infants. *Lancet Infect Dis.* **2014**, *14*, 751–762. [CrossRef]
24. Villamor-Martinez, E.; Fumagalli, M.; Mohammed Rahim, O.; Passera, S.; Cavallaro, G.; Degraeuwe, P.; Mosca, F.; Villamor, E. Chorioamnionitis Is a Risk Factor for Intraventricular Hemorrhage in Preterm Infants: A Systematic Review and Meta-Analysis. *Front. Physiol.* **2018**, *9*, 1253. [CrossRef] [PubMed]
25. Hoyle, E.S.; Patino, F.; Yoxall, C.W. Quality improvement programme to improve compliance with initial respiratory support guideline at preterm birth. *Acta Paediatr.* **2020**, *109*, 943–947. [CrossRef] [PubMed]

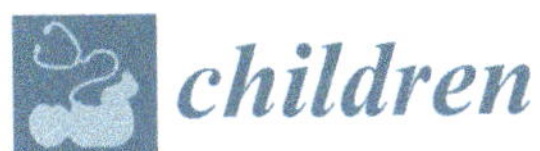

Study Protocol

Efficacy of Intact Cord Resuscitation Compared to Immediate Cord Clamping on Cardiorespiratory Adaptation at Birth in Infants with Isolated Congenital Diaphragmatic Hernia (CHIC)

Kévin Le Duc [1,2,3,*], Sébastien Mur [2,3], Thameur Rakza [2,3], Mohamed Riadh Boukhris [2,3], Céline Rousset [2,3], Pascal Vaast [3,4], Nathalie Westlynk [4], Estelle Aubry [1,3,5], Dyuti Sharma [1,3,5] and Laurent Storme [1,2,3]

[1] ULR2694 Metrics-Perinatal Environment and Health, University of Lille, 59000 Lille, France; estelle.aubry@chru-lille.fr (E.A.); dyuti.sharma@chru-lille.fr (D.S.); laurent.storme@chru-lille.fr (L.S.)

[2] Department of Neonatology, Jeanne de Flandre Hospital, Centre Hospitalier Universitaire de Lille, 59000 Lille, France; sebastien.mur@chru-lille.fr (S.M.); Thameur.RAKZA@chru-lille.fr (T.R.); riadh.boukhris@chru-lille.fr (M.R.B.); Celine.rousset@chru-lille.fr (C.R.)

[3] Center for Rare Disease Congenital Diaphragmatic Hernia, Jeanne de Flandre Hospital, Centre Hospitalier Universitaire de Lille, 59000 Lille, France; pascal.vaast@chru-lille.fr

[4] Department of Obstetrics, Jeanne de Flandre Hospital, Centre Hospitalier Universitaire de Lille, 59000 Lille, France; nathalie.westlynk@chru-lille.fr

[5] Department of Pediatric Surgery, Jeanne de Flandre Hospital, Centre Hospitalier Universitaire de Lille, 59000 Lille, France

* Correspondence: kevin.leduc@chru-lille.fr; Tel.: +33-32-044-6199

Citation: Le Duc, K.; Mur, S.; Rakza, T.; Boukhris, M.R.; Rousset, C.; Vaast, P.; Westlynk, N.; Aubry, E.; Sharma, D.; Storme, L. Efficacy of Intact Cord Resuscitation Compared to Immediate Cord Clamping on Cardiorespiratory Adaptation at Birth in Infants with Isolated Congenital Diaphragmatic Hernia (CHIC). *Children* **2021**, *8*, 339. https://doi.org/10.3390/children8050339

Academic Editor: Simone Pratesi

Received: 31 March 2021
Accepted: 22 April 2021
Published: 26 April 2021

Publisher's Note: MDPI stays neutral with regard to jurisdictional claims in published maps and institutional affiliations.

Abstract: Resuscitation at birth of infants with Congenital Diaphragmatic Hernia (CDH) remains highly challenging because of severe failure of cardiorespiratory adaptation at birth. Usually, the umbilical cord is clamped immediately after birth. Delaying cord clamping while the resuscitation maneuvers are started may: (1) facilitate blood transfer from placenta to baby to augment circulatory blood volume; (2) avoid loss of venous return and decrease in left ventricle filling caused by immediate cord clamping; (3) prevent initial hypoxemia because of sustained uteroplacental gas exchange after birth when the cord is intact. The aim of this trial is to evaluate the efficacy of intact cord resuscitation compared to immediate cord clamping on cardiorespiratory adaptation at birth in infants with isolated CDH. The Congenital Hernia Intact Cord (CHIC) trial is a prospective multicenter open-label randomized controlled trial in two balanced parallel groups. Participants are randomized either immediate cord clamping (the cord will be clamped within the first 15 s after birth) or to intact cord resuscitation group (umbilical cord will be kept intact during the first part of the resuscitation). The primary end-point is the number of infants with APGAR score <4 at 1 min or <7 at 5 min. One hundred eighty participants are expected for this trial. To our knowledge, CHIC is the first study randomized controlled trial evaluating intact cord resuscitation on newborn infant with congenital diaphragmatic hernia. Better cardiorespiratory adaptation is expected when the resuscitation maneuvers are started while the cord is still connected to the placenta.

Keywords: intact cord resuscitation; delivery room resuscitation; congenital diaphragmatic hernia

1. Introduction

Congenital Diaphragmatic Hernia (CDH) is a rare disease (1/3000 pregnancies) caused by diaphragmatic defect with ascension of the abdominal content into the thoracic cavity. Pulmonary consequences of CDH present a broad spectrum of severity [1]. Despite major improvement in neonatal intensive care, mortality and morbidity related to failure of transition at birth remain high with a mortality rate between 20 to 40% [2]. Failure of transition at birth results from persistent pulmonary hypertension (PPHN) and is almost a universal finding in CDH [3,4]. There is an urgent need for additional research in order to promote cardiorespiratory adaptation at birth.

The CDH EURO Consortium proposes intubating newborn infants with CDH immediately after birth to limit PPHN [5]. Treatment in the delivery room is directed at reaching an adequate oxygenation while avoiding high airway pressures. Low peak pressures are given to avoid lung damage to the hypoplastic and contralateral lung [4]. Resuscitation at birth remains highly challenging because of severe failure of cardiorespiratory adaptation at birth. Despite the recommendations, aggressive resuscitation if often applied because the baby is frequently cyanotic and bradycardic as soon as the umbilical cord is sectioned. Pneumothoraces—a marker of barotrauma—can occur early after starting the resuscitation maneuvers and is associated with high mortality rate [6]. A postmortem CDH study has shown that the high mortality in CDH can be partially attributed to pulmonary barotrauma causing damage to hypoplastic lungs [7]. Therefore, the immediate postnatal period of resuscitation represents a window of extreme vulnerability of the baby with CDH, conditioning the short- and long-term outcome.

Traditionally, the umbilical cord is clamped and cut immediately after birth. Clamping the umbilical cord immediately increases systemic peripheral resistance, resulting in an increase in arterial pressure (afterload). However, as the placental circulation receives 30–50% of fetal cardiac output, cord clamping transiently reduces venous return (by 30–50%), which, combined with the increase in afterload, decreases cardiac output [8]. Following cord clamping, umbilical venous return is lost and left ventricular output becomes dependent on pulmonary blood flow, as in adults. Any delay between umbilical cord clamping and the increase in pulmonary blood flow could therefore severely affect left ventricular output and potentially result in organ injury. In CDH infant, increase in pulmonary blood flow is delayed after birth because of PPHN. These changes may significantly impact on cardiac function after clamping of the cord.

In 2015, the International Liaison Committee on Resuscitation (ILCOR) recommended that the cord should not be cut for at least 1 to 3 min after birth in infants not requiring resuscitation [9]. This recommended change in practice is to facilitate blood transfer from placenta to baby to reduce iron deficiency and later anemia in the full-term newborn infant. In the same way, meta-analysis indicate that delayed cord clamping in the preterm infant increases circulating volume and improves blood pressure, reduces the need for blood transfusion, risk of intraventricular hemorrhage and necrotizing enterocolitis [10,11].

The ex-utero intrapartum treatment (EXIT) procedure has been proposed during a variety of surgical procedures, mainly cervical mass resection, performed at birth to secure the fetal airway or ensure successful transition to postnatal environment [12]. The aim of the EXIT procedure is to maintain placental gas exchange while steps are taken to optimize the transition of the newborn infant from fetal to neonatal life.

Preliminary Data Obtained

We have shown in three previous studies in normal newborn lambs and in newborn lambs with PPHN that blood gases did not change 30 min after birth despite lack of breathing compared to the blood gases obtained before birth [13–15].

We also evaluated the safety, feasibility and impacts of intact cord resuscitation (ICR) on cardiorespiratory adaptation at birth in newborn infants with CDH in a prospective pilot study [16].

Resuscitation before cord clamping was possible for all infants in the ICR group. The cord was clamped at 7 ± 3 min after birth. No increase in maternal or neonatal adverse events was observed during the period of ICR.

A multicenter randomized clinical study is required to confirm the benefit of intact cord resuscitation in CDH infants on cardiorespiratory adaptation at birth. To know whether intact cord resuscitation improves initial cardiorespiratory adaptation at birth is a major issue.

2. Materials and Methods

2.1. Objectives

2.1.1. Primary Endpoints

The primary endpoint is the rate of infants with APGAR score < 4 at 1 min or <7 at 5 min.

This primary objective is to show the efficacy of intact cord resuscitation compared to immediate cord clamping on cardiorespiratory adaptation at birth in full term newborn infants with isolated CDH. APGAR score is used to assess cardiorespiratory adaptation at birth. APGAR score is based on clinical assessment of color, heart rate, grimace, muscle tone, and respiratory effort. It is used worldwide by neonatal caregivers, both as a measure of the infant's clinical status as well as a measure of the infant's response to resuscitation. APGAR score can be assessed during resuscitation maneuvers, including intubation. Slight inter-observer variation may exist in intubated baby mainly due to lack of standardization of scoring respiratory effort states. In order to limit inter-observer variability, we will standardize respiratory effort scoring as previously reported [17]. In order to optimize APGAR scoring, each of its five items will be recorded by two observers. A timer is switched on at birth. Apgar will be assessed at 1, 5 and 10 min.

APGAR is universally recognized as a major prognostic variable of neonatal outcome [18]. More specifically, APGAR scoring remains the main early predictor for mortality in isolated CDH infant [19]. Low APGAR score (<7 at 5 min) is associated with an increased risk of death (OR 2.7 (1.9–4)) in a cohort of 2202 infants with CDH.

2.1.2. Secondary Endpoints

The secondary objectives of the studies are as follows:

1. To ensure maternal safety of the procedure, blood loss will be carefully monitored after birth. A graduated collector bag for blood, placed under the woman's buttocks just after delivery of the child, will be used systematically to measure the blood lost through the vagina in the immediate postpartum period. This bag will be left in place at least for 15 min. The following maternal safety endpoints will be assessed:
   - Frequency of postpartum hemorrhage (PPH) defined by blood loss $\geq$ 500 mL;
   - Frequency of severe PPH, defined by measured blood loss $\geq$ 1000 mL;
   - Blood loss volume at 15 min after birth;
   - Total postpartum blood loss volume (at bag removal);

2. To assess the effect of intact cord resuscitation compared to immediate cord clamping on cardiorespiratory adaptation of infants after birth, the following secondary endpoints will be assessed:
   - Frequency of infants with the need for epinephrine administration and/or fluid resuscitation;
   - Frequency of infants with the need for chest compressions;
   - Pre-ductal SpO2, and heart rate at 1, 5, and 10 min after birth: a pulse oxymeter sensor will be placed at the right hand as soon as possible (within the first minute after birth), which then will be connected to a pulse oxymeter;
   - Blood gases and plasma lactate concentration at one hour after birth (H1): these quantitative variables can be considered as objective markers of early cardiorespiratory adaptation at birth.
   - Blood gases, pre- and postductal SpO2, lactate, FiO2 set to obtain preductal SpO2 90–94%, ventilatory parameters (peak inspiratory pressure, respiratory rate), heart rate, blood pressure, and urine output at H1, H24, H48, H72, D7, D28;
   - Volume of fluid resuscitation during the first 24 h;
   - Frequency of infants with the need for vasoactive drugs during the first 24 h;
   - Frequency of infants with the need for pulmonary vasodilator during the first 24 h;
   - Hemoglobin concentration at H24;
   - Echocardiographic parameters (left and right mean blood flow velocities, pulmonary artery pressure) at H6, H24, H48, D7, D28;

3. To assess the effect of intact cord resuscitation compared to immediate cord clamping on infants' mortality and morbidity, we choose to assess the number of free-days from medical support in order to address the effect of mortality on the assessment of morbidity. Because of the randomization process, we can assume that the two groups will be similar in term of severity. In the hypothesis that intact cord resuscitation decreases the mortality, it means that more severe CDH infant may survive, which may in turn increase the apparent morbidity. In case of death, the number of free-days from medical support is zero, which will not modify the number of free-days from medical support in the surviving population. Therefore, the following secondary end-points will be assessed:

    -   Infant mortality rate at 90-day after birth;
    -   Infant morbidity outcomes assessed within the first 90 days after birth:

        o   mechanical ventilation free-days (defined as days alive and free of mechanical ventilation from birth to 90 days),

        o   extracorporeal membranous oxygenation free-days (defined as days alive and free of extracorporeal membranous oxygenation from birth to 90 days)

        o   pulmonary vasodilator treatment free-days (defined as days alive and free of pulmonary vasodilator treatment including inhaled NO, sildenafil, prostacyclin analog, bosentan from birth to 90 days),

        o   O2 supplementation free-days (defined as days alive and free of O2 supplementation including non-invasive respiratory support from birth to 90 days),

        o   parenteral nutrition free-days (defined as days alive and free of parenteral nutrition from birth to 90 days)

        o   Total duration of hospitalization,

4. To assess parental acceptability and psychological impact of starting resuscitation while the cord is intact as compared to the immediate cord clamping group:

    -   Number of refusals to participating with the protocol: the reasons for refusal will be recorded (do not want to participate to a research protocol, to not want to be randomized in the immediate cord clamping group, to not want to be randomized in the intact cord resuscitation group);
    -   Anxiety and depression level assessed by Hospital Anxiety and Depression Scale, HADS. HADS is an auto-questionnaire translated in French, including seven questions to assess anxiety and seven questions to assess depression. HADS questionnaire lasts 3 to 6 min, and is mostly well accepted. Both parents will be requested to answer the questionnaire within the first 3 days after birth, in a calm and neutral room at the maternity ward. Psychologist in charge of the parents will be informed of the results of the test to adapt family support if required;
    -   Semi-structured interviews will be proposed by a psychologist to the parents whatever the issue, at the end of the study period (90 $\pm$ 7 days after birth) to assess their personal experience of the resuscitating period at birth, including both early/delayed cord clamping and close/remote resuscitation maneuvers. The interviews tape recordings will be transcribed and then analyzed using thematic coding. The anonymized data will be independently coded by three researchers and compared for consistency of interpretation. The themes that emerged following the final coding will be used for a qualitative analysis of the parental verbatim;

2.2. Trial Design

This is a prospective multicenter open-label randomized controlled trial in two balanced parallel groups.

2.3. Inclusion Criteria

Antenatal diagnosis of CDH
No severe additional malformation or chromosomal diseases
Full term (>36 weeks gestational age)
No inclusion in another antenatal trial
Written informed consents from the parents
The fetuses which required Fetoscopic Endoluminal Tracheal Occlusion (FETO procedure) will also be included in the study.

2.4. Exclusion Criteria

Preterm birth before 37 weeks gestational age
Other severe malformation(s) or chromosomal diseases
Need for emergency cesarean section ("red code")
Twin pregnancy
Postnatal diagnosis of additional severe malformation(s) or chromosomal diseases

2.5. Study Organization

After assessing the inclusion and exclusion criteria, the parents will be informed of the study protocol and the intact cord resuscitation procedure (between 22- and 36-weeks gestational age). The written parental consents are requested before 37 weeks gestational age. A web-based randomization with electronic case-report form (eCRF) system is performed at admission for delivery at the maternity ward. Prenatal o/e LHR on ultrasounds and lung volumetry on fetal MRI allow to classify patients in according the severity of the CDH (mild, moderate, severe and extremely severe) [20,21]. Randomization is stratified according to center, and four antenatal severity subgroups defined by ultrasound lung-to-head ratio Observed/Expected and liver position (Extreme <15%, Severe 15–25%, Moderate 25–45%, and Mild >45%).

The infants with CDH will be included in the study and randomized in one of the two groups. Severity subgroups is considered as a stratified factor in randomization. A dynamic randomization procedure using the Pocock and Simon minimization method is used [22]. Whatever the group of randomization, the national guidelines [23,24] for resuscitation maneuvers in the delivery room will be applied similarly in both groups. Except the timing of cord clamping, the overall management including the resuscitation maneuvers in the delivery room (intact cord resuscitation group) or resuscitation room (early cord clamping group), and organization of the follow-up will be similar in both groups. In particular, the main resuscitation maneuvers at birth are:

- The newborn infant should be intubated routinely without bag and mask ventilation, with an endotracheal tube 3.5 mm;
- Ventilation in the delivery room should be done with a peak pressure below 25 cmH2O, and an initial FiO2 = 1;
- The goal of treatment in the delivery room is achieving heart rate > 120 beats/min and increasing preductal SpO2 or achieving acceptable preductal SpO2 targets between 80 and 95%;
- An oro- or nasogastric tube with continuous or intermittent suction should be placed;
- Group 1: Immediate cord clamping with transfer to the resuscitation room

In the immediate cord clamping group, the cord will be clamped within the first 20 s after birth and the infant will be transferred to the resuscitation room. The newborn infant will be intubated and mechanically ventilated as quickly as possible on the resuscitation table as recommended in the Programme National de Soins. After cardiorespiratory stabilization (heart rate > 120/min, increasing preductal O2 saturation or achieving acceptable preductal SpO2 targets between 80 and 95%), the infant will be transferred to the neonatal intensive care unit (NICU). Oxytocin is infused to the mother as recommended in the local protocol (usually just after birth or cord clamping).

- Group 2: Intact cord resuscitation with resuscitation maneuvers performed on a dedicated trolley placed close to the mother

In the intact cord resuscitation group, the umbilical cord will be kept intact during the initial phase of the resuscitation. The infant will be placed on a specifically designed compact trolley with a warmed platform, suitable for commencing resuscitation between the mother's legs in case of vaginal birth or near the operating table beside the mother in case of cesarean section. This trolley will be fully equipped for resuscitation, including a suction device, gas flowmeter/blender, ventilator, and monitoring system. Its height can be adjusted to position the infant close to the maternal perineum. The infant will be intubated and mechanically ventilated on this trolley; special care will be taken to prevent stretching, compression, or kinking of the cord. The cord will be clamped after cardiorespiratory stabilization will be obtained (heart rate > 120/min, increasing preductal O2 saturation or achieving acceptable preductal SpO2 targets between 80 and 95%) or in case of spontaneous placental expulsion. Oxytocin is infused to the mother just after cord clamping. The infant will be then transferred to the NICU. See Figure 1 "Study organization".

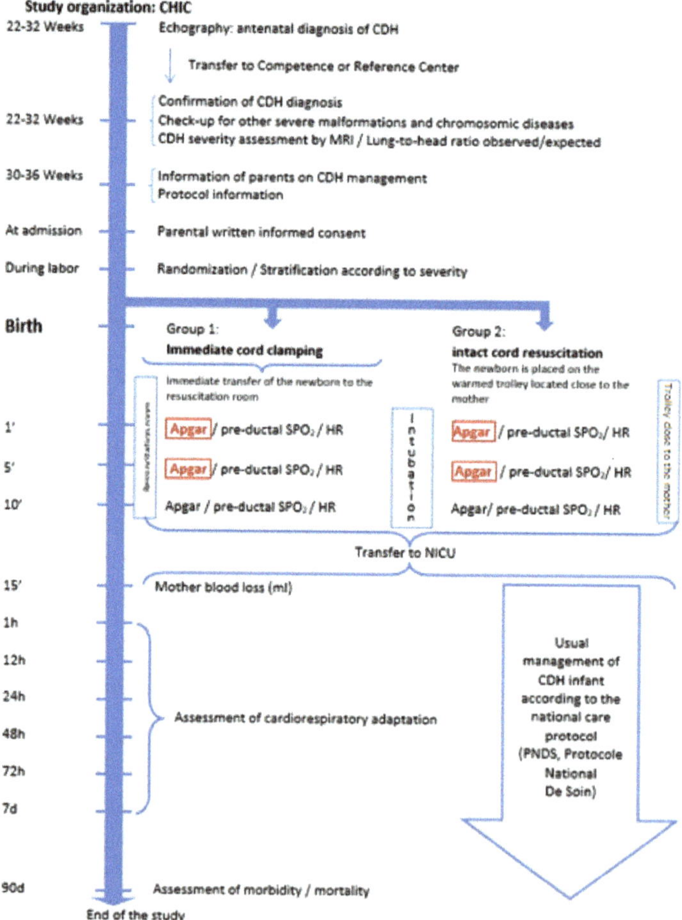

Figure 1. Study organization. Congenital Diaphragmatic Hernia (CDH); Congenital Hernia Intact Cord (CHIC); Blood oxygen saturation (SpO2); Heart Rate (HR); Neonatal Intensive Care Unit (NICU).

2.6. Interventions

Except the timing of cord clamping, the national guidelines will be applied during the course of the prenatal and postnatal management.

Some differences with usual care during implementation of the protocol are as follows:

- Here is a photograph of the trolley (LifeStart, Inspiration Healthcare, Great Britain) (Figure 2):

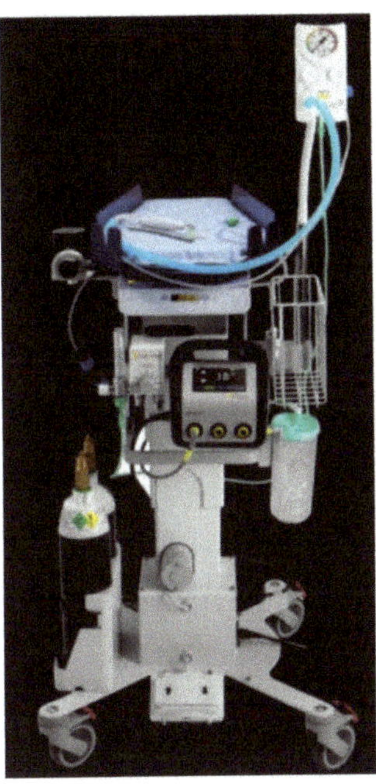

Figure 2. The resuscitation table Lifestart is easily maneuverable, with ergonomic top for placement of the baby. It is equipped with a neonatal warming system, a built-in timer that tracks clamping delay, and a suction device. The baby is warmed from under the patient, ensuring that there is no impediment to resuscitation maneuvers. The electrically operated raising and lowering mechanism allows the nursing platform to be easily positioned at the optimal height for each individual situation and adjusted as necessary. All the resuscitation equipment can be positioned close to the mother and adapted for all types of delivery: natural; assisted; or caesarean section.

- In both groups, although APGAR score is routinely assessed in every baby at 1 and 5 mn, special care will be taken to optimize scoring taken into account the fact that most infants with CDH are intubated at 5 min. APGAR score can be assessed during resuscitation maneuvers, including intubation. Slight inter-observer variation may exist in intubated baby mainly due to lack of standardization of scoring respiratory effort states [22]. In order to limit inter-observer variability, we will standardize respiratory effort scoring as previously reported [22]:
- an infant who is apneic and requires intubation and ventilation should receive the minimum value of 0 for respiratory effort;
- an infant who requires artificial ventilation at birth due to irregular or shallow ventilation should score 1;
- To assess whether an artificially ventilated infant is apnoeic or not, ventilation should be stopped briefly, when possible, to check for the presence of spontaneous respiratory movements (apneic, score = 0; irregular or shallow ventilation, score 1; spontaneous effective ventilation, score 2).

- Preductal SpO2 and heart rate are routinely assessed in every baby with CDH. They will be recorded at 1, 5 and 10 min after birth in both groups.
- Blood gases and lactate concentration are routinely assessed in every baby with CDH. These parameters will be recorded at H1, H12, H24, H48, H72, D7, D28, in both groups. Compared with usual care, no additional blood samples are required for the protocol;
- In both groups, although noninvasive echocardiography is routinely assessed in every baby with CDH, left and right mean blood flow velocities, pulmonary artery pressure will be recorded at H6, H24, H48, D7, D28. Compared with usual care, no additional echocardiography is required for the protocol;
- Acceptability by the parents and psychological impact of intact cord resuscitation will be assessed using a questionnaire and a semi-directive interview.

2.7. Criteria for Discontinuation of the Procedure

The healthcare providers (obstetrician, midwives, anesthetist, and pediatrician) in charge of the baby or the mother may stop the procedure—i.e., clamp the cord—if they judge it is required for the safety of the patient. The reason for stopping the procedure and the timing at cord clamping will be recorded. In that case, the patient is not excluded from the study and the variable is recorded as planned in the protocol. The patient data are analyzed according to intention to treat principle.

The follow-up of the infants is planned till the age of 3 months (90 days), corresponding to the last visit. If the patient is transferred in another hospital, the variable will be recorded till the age of 3 months.

2.8. Sample Size Calculation

The primary objective is to show the superiority of intact cord resuscitation (experimental group) compared to immediate cord clamping (control group) to improve cardiorespiratory adaptation at birth of CDH infant. The primary endpoint is defined as the rate of infants with low APGAR score, defined by a APGAR score < 4 at 1 min or <7 at 5 min of life. On the basis of literature, we expected that 37% of CDH infant in control arm will have a low APGAR score. To show a 50% relative reduction (corresponding to a rate of 18.5% in experimental group), with a type I error of 5% (two-sided test), and a power of 80%, we calculated that 90 subjects (mother/infant) per group are needed, which means a total of 180 subjects.

2.9. Statistical Analysis Plan

Statistical analyses will be independently performed by the Biostatistics Department of University of Lille under the responsibility of Professor Alain Duhamel. For the data analysis, statisticians will be unaware of the treatment group allocation. Data will be analyzed using the SAS software (SAS Institute Inc., Cary, NC, USA) and all statistical tests will be performed with a two-tailed alpha risk of 0.05. All analyses will be performed in all randomized patients based on their original group of randomizations, according to the intention-to-treat principle. No interim analysis will be performed. A detailed statistical analysis plan will be written and finalized prior to the database lock.

Baseline characteristics will be described for each group. Quantitative variables will be expressed as mean (standard deviation), or median (interquartile range) for non-Gaussian distribution. Categorical variables will be expressed as frequencies and percentages. Normality of distribution will be assessed graphically and using the Shapiro–Wilk test.

2.10. Data Safety Monitoring Board

The Data and Safety Monitoring Board (DSMB) is an independent consultative board asked to express an opinion to the sponsor of the study on the benefit/risk ratio and the management of the clinical trial.

A DSMB will be set up, composed of the following members, at least: two pediatricians, two obstetricians, one anesthetist, and one methodologist.

Its members will not participate in the study and will be independent from the investigation centers. They will be nominated by the sponsor of the study and will participate as volunteers in the respect of confidentiality of the data.

The DSMB will analyze the management of the study as well as its benefit/risk exposure and might recommend to stop the study in certain circumstances:

- If the number of Serious Adverse Event (SAE) within the first 24 h after birth is twice higher in the "intact cord resuscitation" group after the inclusion of 30 patients,
- If the DSMB judges that a reported SAE caused by the procedure requires to stop the study,
- If inclusion rate is less than 25% of the total inclusion objectives, 24 months after starting the inclusion in the study. The board will meet after the inclusion of 30, 90 and 150 patients, to address those points, but it could be summoned on other circumstances:
- If a mother's death occurs within three months after she gave birth to her child,
- At the request of any PI involved in the study.

3. Results

Presently, 11 centers are participating to the study: two additional centers are expected to include CDH infants. The first center started enrolling patients for 6 months. At the present time, 10 patients have been recruited. For now, parental consents have been obtained in all cases. Recruitment is expected to be completed by December 2023.

4. Discussion

Resuscitation at birth of infants with congenital diaphragmatic hernia remains highly challenging because of severe failure of cardiorespiratory adaptation at birth.

The traditional approach in the delivery room is immediate cord clamping followed by intubation. Initiating resuscitation prior to umbilical cord clamping (UCC) may support this transition, to avoid the loss of venous return and decrease in left ventricle filling caused by cord clamping, ideally increase in pulmonary blood flow should precede cord clamping. This would enable pulmonary venous return to replace umbilical venous return as the primary source for left ventricle preload and to minimize swings in left ventricular output caused by cord clamping. In infants with CDH, the cord is clamped while the pulmonary blood flow is still low.

Evidence indicates that utero-placental gas exchange continues after birth when the cord is intact. A previous experimental study in newborn lambs showed that heart rates and right ventricle output were markedly decreased within 120 s of cord clamping. In contrast, if umbilical cord clamping was delayed until after ventilation had commenced, these large changes in heart rate, arterial pressures and flows were greatly reduced, resulting in a much more stable cardiovascular transition after birth [25,26]. We hypothesize that delayed cord clamping allows time for the infant to aerate its lungs and increase pulmonary blood flow before venous return from the placental circulation is lost.

Preliminary study has demonstrated the feasibility of intact cord resuscitation. Starting mechanical ventilation of the infant newborn with congenital diaphragmatic hernia before clamping the cord allowed a potential benefit to improved blood pressure at 1 h of life compared to those resuscitated traditionally [27].

Lefebvre et al. demonstrated that Intact cord resuscitation was associated with higher APGAR scores at 1 and 5 min after birth. The pH was higher and the plasma lactate concentration was significantly lower at one hour after birth in the intact cord resuscitation than in the immediate cord clamp group (pH = 7.17 ± 0.1 vs. 7.08 ± 0.2; lactate = 3.6 ± 2 vs. 6.6 ± 4 mmol/L, $p < 0.05$). Mean blood pressure was significantly higher in the intact cord resuscitation than in the immediate cord clamp group at H1 (52 ± 7 vs. 42 ± 7 mmHg), H6 (47 ± 3 vs. 40 ± 5 mmHg) and H12 (44 ± 2 vs. 39 ± 3 mmHg) ($p < 0.05$). Therefore, commencing resuscitation and initiating ventilation while the infant is still attached to the placenta is feasible in infants with CDH. The procedure is safe, and may support the cardiorespiratory transition at birth in infants with CDH [16].

To our knowledge, CHIC trial is the first prospective multicenter randomized controlled trial to assess the impact of delayed cord clamping during resuscitation of newborn infant with congenital diaphragmatic hernia. Future publication on the primary and secondary results of the CHIC trial study will make a substantial contribution to this important orientation of research and the results will provide clear evidence on the impact of delayed cord clamping during resuscitation of the newborn infant with congenital diaphragmatic hernia.

Author Contributions: Conceptualization, L.S., T.R. and S.M.; Funding acquisition: L.S.; Project Administration, C.R.; writing—original draft preparation, K.L.D.; writing—review and editing, L.S., K.L.D., C.R. and S.M.; Investigation, S.M., K.L.D., M.R.B., L.S., T.R., P.V., N.W., E.A. and D.S. All authors have read and agreed to the published version of the manuscript.

Funding: This research received funding from DGOS (the French national medical and care ministry), grant number PHRC-18-0234.

Institutional Review Board Statement: This project was reviewed and managed by the Lille's University Public Hospital Review Board and is conducted according to the guidelines of the Declaration of Helsinki and received: CPP (Ethics Committee) approval on 09/03/2019, ANSM authorization on 07/30/2019, CNIL attestation on 06/24/2019 and contracted insurance on 05/14/2019 (Protocol code: IDRCB #3019-A01030-57). The Clinical Trials.gov identifier of this study is: NCT04429750. Recruitment starting date: October 2020. Trial status: Recruiting. Recruitment began on September 2020 and is expected to be completed September 2023.

Informed Consent Statement: For this research, a written informed consent is obtained from all subjects involved in the study.

Acknowledgments: We acknowledge the Data Safety Monitoring Board of this study; EuroCare-France for its participation and collaboration; implication and contribution of team members of all the participating hospitals including: obstetricians, anesthetists, pediatricians, surgeons, clinical research data set technicians. Florence Nosal for her help in funding acquisition. Eloise Dewuite for her help in project administration. Alain Duhamel and Julien Labreuche for their help in methodologic design of the study. Florence Flamein for her help in project management and investigation. Principal investigators engaged in this study: Beuchee Alain, Boubred Farid, Cambonie Gilles, Claris Olivier, Flamant Cyril, Kermorvant Elsa, Mokhtari Mostafa, Savey Baptiste, Tandonnet Olivier, Tourneux Pierre.

Conflicts of Interest: The authors declare no conflict of interest.

References

1. Skari, H.; Bjornland, K.; Haugen, G.; Egeland, T.; Emblem, R. Congenital Diaphragmatic Hernia: A Meta-Analysis of Mortality Factors. *J. Pediatric Surg.* **2000**, *35*, 1187–1197. [CrossRef] [PubMed]
2. Congenital Diaphragmatic Hernia Study Group; Morini, F.; Valfrè, L.; Capolupo, I.; Lally, K.P.; Lally, P.A.; Bagolan, P. Congenital Diaphragmatic Hernia: Defect Size Correlates with Developmental Defect. *J. Pediatric Surg.* **2013**, *48*, 1177–1182. [CrossRef] [PubMed]
3. Storme, L.; Aubry, E.; Rakza, T.; Houeijeh, A.; Debarge, V.; Tourneux, P.; Deruelle, P.; Pennaforte, T. Pathophysiology of Persistent Pulmonary Hypertension of the Newborn: Impact of the Perinatal Environment. *Arch. Cardiovasc. Dis.* **2013**, *106*, 169–177. [CrossRef] [PubMed]
4. Bohn, D. Congenital Diaphragmatic Hernia. *Am. J. Respir. Crit. Care Med.* **2002**, *166*, 911–915. [CrossRef]
5. Snoek, K.G.; Reiss, I.K.M.; Greenough, A.; Capolupo, I.; Urlesberger, B.; Wessel, L.; Storme, L.; Deprest, J.; Schaible, T.; van Heijst, A.; et al. Standardized Postnatal Management of Infants with Congenital Diaphragmatic Hernia in Europe: The CDH EURO Consortium Consensus—2015 Update. *Neonatology* **2016**, *110*, 66–74. [CrossRef]
6. Usui, N.; Nagata, K.; Hayakawa, M.; Okuyama, H.; Kanamori, Y.; Takahashi, S.; Inamura, N.; Taguchi, T. Pneumothoraces As a Fatal Complication of Congenital Diaphragmatic Hernia in the Era of Gentle Ventilation. *Eur. J. Pediatric Surg.* **2013**, *24*, 031–038. [CrossRef]
7. Sakurai, Y.; Azarow, K.; Cutz, E.; Messineo, A.; Pearl, R.; Bohn, D. Pulmonary Barotrauma in Congenital Diaphragmatic Hernia: A Clinicopathological Correlation. *J. Pediatric Surg.* **1999**, *34*, 1813–1817. [CrossRef]

8.   Crossley, K.J.; Allison, B.J.; Polglase, G.R.; Morley, C.J.; Davis, P.G.; Hooper, S.B. Dynamic Changes in the Direction of Blood Flow through the Ductus Arteriosus at Birth: Blood Flow through the Ductus Arteriosus at Birth. *J. Physiol.* **2009**, *587*, 4695–4704. [CrossRef]

9.   Wyckoff, M.H.; Aziz, K.; Escobedo, M.B.; Kapadia, V.S.; Kattwinkel, J.; Perlman, J.M.; Simon, W.M.; Weiner, G.M.; Zaichkin, J.G. Part 13: Neonatal Resuscitation: 2015 American Heart Association Guidelines Update for Cardiopulmonary Resuscitation and Emergency Cardiovascular Care. *Circulation* **2015**, *132*, S543–S560. [CrossRef]

10.   Rabe, H.; Gyte, G.M.; Díaz-Rossello, J.L.; Duley, L. Effect of Timing of Umbilical Cord Clamping and Other Strategies to Influence Placental Transfusion at Preterm Birth on Maternal and Infant Outcomes. *Cochrane Database Syst. Rev.* **2019**. [CrossRef]

11.   Fogarty, M.; Osborn, D.A.; Askie, L.; Seidler, A.L.; Hunter, K.; Lui, K.; Simes, J.; Tarnow-Mordi, W. Delayed vs Early Umbilical Cord Clamping for Preterm Infants: A Systematic Review and Meta-Analysis. *Am. J. Obstet. Gynecol.* **2018**, *218*, 1–18. [CrossRef]

12.   Cass, D.L.; Olutoye, O.O.; Cassady, C.I.; Zamora, I.J.; Ivey, R.T.; Ayres, N.A.; Olutoye, O.A.; Lee, T.C. EXIT-to-Resection for Fetuses with Large Lung Masses and Persistent Mediastinal Compression near Birth. *J. Pediatric Surg.* **2013**, *48*, 138–144. [CrossRef]

13.   Houeijeh, A.; Tourneux, P.; Mur, S.; Aubry, E.; Viard, R.; Sharma, D.; Storme, L. Lung Liquid Clearance in Preterm Lambs Assessed by Magnetic Resonance Imaging. *Pediatric Res.* **2017**, *82*, 114–121. [CrossRef]

14.   Viard, R.; Tourneux, P.; Storme, L.; Girard, J.-M.; Betrouni, N.; Rousseau, J. Magnetic Resonance Imaging Spatial and Time Study of Lung Water Content in Newborn Lamb: Methods and Preliminary Results. *Investig. Radiol.* **2008**, *43*, 470–480. [CrossRef]

15.   Jaillard, S.; Elbaz, F.; Bresson-Just, S.; Riou, Y.; Houfflin-Debarge, V.; Rakza, T.; Larrue, B.; Storme, L. Pulmonary Vasodilator Effects of Norepinephrine during the Development of Chronic Pulmonary Hypertension in Neonatal Lambs. *Br. J. Anaesth.* **2004**, *93*, 818–824. [CrossRef]

16.   Lefebvre, C.; Rakza, T.; Weslinck, N.; Vaast, P.; Houfflin-debarge, V.; Mur, S.; Storme, L. Feasibility and Safety of Intact Cord Resuscitation in Newborn Infants with Congenital Diaphragmatic Hernia (CDH). *Resuscitation* **2017**, *120*, 20–25. [CrossRef]

17.   Lopriore, E.; van Burk, G.F.; Walther, F.J.; de Beaufort, A.J. Correct Use of the Apgar Score for Resuscitated and Intubated Newborn Babies: Questionnaire Study. *BMJ* **2004**, *329*, 143–144. [CrossRef]

18.   Natarajan, G.; Pappas, A.; Shankaran, S. Outcomes in Childhood Following Therapeutic Hypothermia for Neonatal Hypoxic-Ischemic Encephalopathy (HIE). *Semin. Perinatol.* **2016**, *40*, 549–555. [CrossRef]

19.   Bent, D.P.; Nelson, J.; Kent, D.M.; Jen, H.C. Population-Based Validation of a Clinical Prediction Model for Congenital Diaphragmatic Hernias. *J. Pediatrics* **2018**, *201*, 160–165. [CrossRef]

20.   Jani, J.C.; Benachi, A.; Nicolaides, K.H.; Allegaert, K.; Gratacós, E.; Mazkereth, R.; Matis, J.; Tibboel, D.; Van Heijst, A.; Storme, L.; et al. Prenatal Prediction of Neonatal Morbidity in Survivors with Congenital Diaphragmatic Hernia: A Multicenter Study. *Ultrasound Obs. Gynecol.* **2009**, *33*, 64–69. [CrossRef]

21.   Dütemeyer, V.; Cordier, A.-G.; Cannie, M.M.; Bevilacqua, E.; Huynh, V.; Houfflin-Debarge, V.; Verpillat, P.; Olivier, C.; Benachi, A.; Jani, J.C. Prenatal Prediction of Postnatal Survival in Fetuses with Congenital Diaphragmatic Hernia Using MRI: Lung Volume Measurement, Signal Intensity Ratio, and Effect of Experience. *J. Matern. Fetal Neonatal Med.* **2020**, 1–9. [CrossRef] [PubMed]

22.   Pocock, S.J.; Simon, R. Sequential Treatment Assignment with Balancing for Prognostic Factors in the Controlled Clinical Trial. *Biometrics* **1975**, *31*, 103–115. [CrossRef] [PubMed]

23.   Storme, L.; Boubnova, J.; Mur, S.; Pognon, L.; Sharma, D.; Aubry, E.; Sfeir, R.; Vaast, P.; Rakza, T.; Benachi, A.; et al. Review Shows That Implementing a Nationwide Protocol for Congenital Diaphragmatic Hernia Was a Key Factor in Reducing Mortality and Morbidity. *Acta Paediatr.* **2018**, *107*, 1131–1139. [CrossRef] [PubMed]

24.   *Hernie de Coupole Diaphragmatique*; Haute Autorité de Santé: Saint-Denis, France, 2020.

25.   Bhatt, S.; Alison, B.J.; Wallace, E.M.; Crossley, K.J.; Gill, A.W.; Kluckow, M.; Pas, A.B.T.; Morley, C.J.; Polglase, G.R.; Hooper, S.B. Delaying cord clamping until ventilation onset improves cardiovascular function at birth in preterm lambs. *J. Physiol.* **2013**, *591*, 2113–2126. [CrossRef] [PubMed]

26.   Hooper, S.B.; Binder-Heschl, C.; Polglase, G.R.; Gill, A.W.; Kluckow, M.; Wallace, E.M.; Blank, D.; Pas, A.B.T. The timing of umbilical cord clamping at birth: physiological considerations. *Matern. Health Neonatol. Perinatol.* **2016**, *2*, 4. [CrossRef] [PubMed]

27.   Foglia, E.; Ades, A.; Hedrick, H.L.; Rintoul, N.; Munson, D.A.; Moldenhauer, J.; Gebb, J.; Serletti, B.; Chaudhary, A.; Weinberg, D.D.; et al. Initiating resuscitation before umbilical cord clamping in infants with congenital diaphragmatic hernia: a pilot feasibility trial. *Arch. Dis. Child. Fetal Neonatal Ed.* **2020**, *105*, 322–326. [CrossRef] [PubMed]

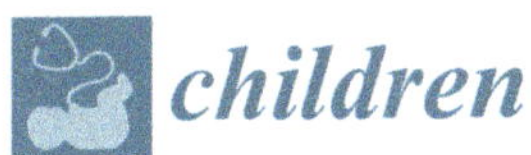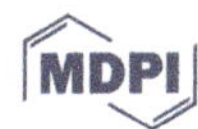

Review

The Use of Foetal Doppler Ultrasound to Determine the Neonatal Heart Rate Immediately after Birth: A Systematic Review

David Hutchon 

Industry and Innovation Research Institute, Sheffield Hallam University, Sheffield S1 1WB, UK; david.hutchon@student.shu.ac.uk

Abstract: Determining the neonatal heart rate immediately after birth is unsatisfactory. Auscultation is inaccurate and provides no documented results. The use of foetal Doppler ultrasound has been recognised as a possible method of determining the neonatal heart rate after birth over the last nine years. This review includes all published studies of this approach, looking at accuracy, speed of results, and practical application of the approach. Precordial Doppler ultrasound has been shown to be as accurate as ECG and more accurate than oximetry for the neonatal heart rate, and provides quicker results than either ECG or oximetry. There is the potential for a much improved determination and documentation of the neonatal heart rate using this approach.

Keywords: neonatal; heart rate; resuscitation; Doppler; precordial

Citation: Hutchon, D. The Use of Foetal Doppler Ultrasound to Determine the Neonatal Heart Rate Immediately after Birth: A Systematic Review. *Children* **2022**, *9*, 717. https://doi.org/10.3390/children9050717

Academic Editor: Joaquim M. B. Pinheiro

Received: 6 April 2022
Accepted: 12 May 2022
Published: 13 May 2022

Publisher's Note: MDPI stays neutral with regard to jurisdictional claims in published maps and institutional affiliations.

1. Introduction

During labour, the main parameter for determining the health of the foetus is heart rate (HR). After birth, when the newborn baby can be observed, heart rate is still a major measure of health—especially in a compromised neonate who is not breathing, crying, or moving. The neonatal branch of the International Liaison Committee on Resuscitation recommends that the heart rate of the newborn baby be determined within the first minute after birth. Heart rate determines the level of care required and any interventions. Auscultation is recommended for routine measurement of the heart rate, which needs to be determined quickly and accurately, since there are specific thresholds for intervention defined by the neonatal heart rate [1].

Determining the heart rate by auscultation requires the number of heartbeats heard to be counted over a known interval of time. The interval needs to be short—6 s or 10 s is recommended—so as to quickly obtain the estimated rate in beats per minute. In healthy neonates, auscultation provides a satisfactory estimate of the heart rate as determined by an ECG, but in a compromised neonate, in a noisy birth room and with weak heart sounds, this may not be the case [2]. Furthermore, the heart rate is undocumented in real time, and there is no opportunity to review the result.

For these reasons, other approaches to determine the heart rate have been sought. Oximetry technology is widespread, reliable, and low-cost. It is the standard for determining the health of neonates. ECG technology is also widespread, and increasingly reliable and low-cost. Both of these technologies take time to apply, and may be difficult after the neonate is placed in a polythene bag—routine care in preterm neonates to reduce the risk of hypothermia. Both of these technologies can readily record and document the heart rate for later review.

A more satisfactory method for routine use to determine the neonatal heart rate at birth is required. Doppler ultrasound is the routine method for monitoring the foetal heart rate. Ultrasound readily passes through the maternal tissues, and the frequency of the reflected sound is altered by the movements of the heart. Heart valve movements are rapid, and result in the major Doppler effects. Foetal heart sounds are familiar to all midwives and obstetricians. The strength of the sound is correlated with the speed of the tissue movement. The heart rate can be determined through an electronic algorithm, or by the clinical assessment of counting over a measured time. The safety of Doppler ultrasound is fully established, with its use in millions of pregnancies over the last 50 years.

Recently, the possibility of this well-established technology used for the foetal heart rate has been explored for use in determining the neonatal heart rate, and the use of Doppler ultrasound forms the basis of this systematic review.

2. Materials and Methods

A literature search using the Medline database with the search terms "neonatal", "doppler", and "heart rate" in the title showed 8 publications; 2 were excluded as not relevant, and a further paper was a review with no new data. A second Medline search using the terms "neonatal", "heart rate", and "resuscitation" in the title identified 24 results. From this, one further paper was identified that described the use of Doppler ultrasound for determination of the neonatal heart rate under "novel techniques". Additional published articles were obtained by manually searching the references in the above publications (Table 1).

Table 1. Human studies included in the review.

Study	Study Design	Comparisons
Zanardo and Parotto (2019) [3]	Observational study of 102 newborns (43 preterm) and 21 requiring resuscitation	ECG vs. 3 MHz Doppler
Shimabukuro et al. (2017) [4]	Prospective cross-sectional study of 33 term neonates at elective caesarean section	ECG vs. 3 MHz Doppler
Agrawal et al. (2021) [5]	Prospective multicentre study, 131 healthy neonates > 34 weeks	ECG vs. 2 MHz Doppler
Goenka et al. (2013) [6]	Prospective study of 92 stable newborns > 37 weeks, 1–8 min after birth	ECG and pulse oximetry vs. 3 MHz Doppler
Kayama et al. (2020) [7]	Prospective study of 102 newborns up to 72 h after birth, 21 during resuscitation, from 23 weeks to term gestation	ECG vs. 3 MHz Doppler

3. Results

Eleven publications were identified as possibly relevant (Table 2). One study by Dyson et al. describing the use of vascular Doppler of the aorta to determine the neonatal heart rate [8], as well as another by Lemke et al. [9] measuring blood flow of the umbilical stump, were excluded (Table 3). A review paper containing no new original data was excluded [2]. Of the remaining studies, five were in human subjects and two in piglets. One excluded study referred to the use of precordial Doppler at birth in the text, but provided no data [10].

Agrawal et al. and Kayama et al. included a range of both healthy and asphyxiated neonates at term or preterm [5,7]. Zanardo et al. [3], Shimabukuro et al. [4], and Goenka et al [6]. focused on healthy neonates. Of the two animal studies, one was in healthy newborn piglets [11], while the other was in asphyxiated piglets [12]. These studies were not included in the data analysis, but are included in the Discussion, for the reasons explained.

Table 2. Human studies included in the review.

Study	Heart Rate Accuracy	Interval from Application to Display
Zanardo and Parotto (2019) [3]	Good correlation between Doppler and pulse oximetry	Mean interval of 3 s for Doppler vs. 5.2 s for ECG
Shimabukuro et al. (2017) [4]	Good correlation between Doppler and ECG	5.6 s for Doppler vs. 5.2 s for ECG
Agrawal et al. (2021) [5]	Mean of 152 for Doppler vs. 161 for ECG	Significantly quicker for Doppler
Goenka et al. (2013) [6]	Good correlation between Doppler and ECG	Equivalent time to ECG and quicker than oximetry
Kayama et al. (2020) [7]	Good correlation between Doppler and ECG. A crying, moving baby may make Doppler measurements difficult	Mean of 5 s for Doppler vs. 10 s for ECG

Table 3. Excluded studies.

Dyson J et al. (2017) [8]
Lemke RP et al. (2011) [9]
Kevat AC et al. (2017) [2]
Katheria AC et al. (2017) [10]

The foetal Doppler machines used in the studies were either 2 or 3 MHz transducers. All were handheld transducers placed over the neonatal precordium with a sound output and a digital heart rate display. The gold standard for the heart rate in the studies was the electrocardiogram (ECG), and in addition, pulse oximetry was measured in one study. All studies showed a satisfactory correlation of the displayed heart rate between Doppler and the gold standard.

The time taken after application of the Doppler probe for a digital heart rate display was quite variable between the studies, but was less than or equivalent to the time taken for the ECG to display a heart rate.

In one study, the authors found that the Doppler ultrasound did not function well with crying and moving babies [7].

4. Discussion

The current clinical approach for determining and documenting the heart rate of a baby immediately after birth is not satisfactory. It is inaccurate, and it is usually more than one minute after birth before the heart rate is obtained [2]. To guide further intervention in compromised neonates, the attendant needs to know whether predefined HR targets have been reached. The effectiveness of positive pressure ventilation (PPV) is determined by an increase in the neonatal HR.

The findings from the piglet studies are included in this review because they demonstrate that the Doppler approach can still detect the heart rate even in very preterm neonates of 500 g—the same weight as a typical newborn piglet. Morina et al. also showed that Doppler ultrasound worked satisfactorily in severely asphyxiated piglets [12]. Hutchon showed the heart rate could be determined and documented within seconds after birth even in these tiny animals [11].

4.1. Accuracy and Time Taken to Obtain the Heart Rate

Auscultation is the recommended mode to determine the initial heart rate in newborns by ILCOR [1]. It takes no significant amount of time to place the stethoscope on the neonate's chest. However, thereafter, methods for getting an accurate heart rate are unsatisfactory. Auscultation is intermittent, and heard by only one clinician, who has to count the number of heartbeats over a fixed time period. Inevitably, this method has limited accuracy, and is undocumented for later review and audit. Background noise in the delivery room may further interfere with the audible heart sounds—especially with the low-level heart sounds of a compromised or preterm neonate.

The application of an ECG (2–3 electrodes) or pulse oximeter takes considerably longer than the application of a stethoscope. The application of the Doppler, however, should be equivalent to applying the stethoscope.

The long latency period of 1 to 2 min before a reliable signal display is obtained from the ECG and PO is a serious shortcoming, as this long interval may interfere with optimal care of the neonate during the first minutes after birth. Some of this time is taken to apply the oximeter sensor or ECG electrodes—longer if three rather than two electrodes are necessary (depending on the equipment being used).

The ECG is considered the gold standard for the accurate measurement of the heart rate (with the previous qualification). Algorithms within the equipment determine the interval between two QRS complexes to measure the heart rate. There are similar algorithms within the Doppler and oximetry electronics. The time taken to display a result, and the result's precision, are therefore very dependent upon the make, design, and age of the Doppler, ECG, or oximetry electronics, but all equipment used in these studies in the last 10 years can be considered satisfactory.

4.2. Safety

All four methods of neonatal heart rate have an established safety record. Intrapartum monitoring (CTG) with Doppler ultrasound has been used in millions of births throughout the world over the last 30 or more years. The ultrasound gel used to facilitate the transmission of ultrasound from the transducer to the neonatal chest is routinely used in colour Doppler examination of the neonatal heart, and there have been no adverse effects reported. However there have been concerns about the ECG electrodes—especially when applied for longer than a few minutes—causing pain or injury to the newborn's skin [5].

Hypothermia is a concern at birth with the exposed wet newborn skin. Babies are therefore routinely dried and wrapped in towels, although an exposed newborn baby can be safely cared for under an infrared lamp present on the neonatal resuscitation trolley. After application of the ECG electrodes and pulse oximeter, the baby can be covered. Application of the precordial Doppler, on the other hand, requires exposure of the chest. However, exposure of the chest may also be necessary during resuscitation to check for the entry of air to the lungs, or to observe chest movements. For a preterm neonate placed in a polythene wrap to reduce the risk of hypothermia, the Doppler ultrasound will still function through the polythene.

Auscultation requires the head of the stethoscope to be placed on the neonate's chest with sufficient pressure to provide good contact with the neonatal skin, but avoiding any excessive pressure that could interfere with chest's expansion during breathing. In practice, avoiding excessive pressure may be quite difficult. The same limitation applies to the precordial handheld Doppler.

4.3. Resuscitation

In a baby who is breathing, crying, or moving, determining the heart rate immediately after birth is not a priority, and Kayama et al. showed that the application of Doppler ultrasound is sometimes difficult in these babies [7]. However, auscultation is likely to be just as limited, and the precise heart rate is of little importance in these healthy babies. It is in hypotonic, apnoeic neonates—likely to require assistance to transition from placental to pulmonary respiration—that there is some urgency to know the heart rate, and whether it is increasing or decreasing [13]. Knowledge of the accurate heart rate of a hypotonic, apnoeic neonate by the whole resuscitation team is important. Ideally, this needs to be a continuous result from soon after birth, and fully documented for subsequent case review. If the Doppler heart sounds are heard by the whole team, they can make estimates of the rate and whether or not it is increasing. Some estimates of the strength of the cardiac contraction may be possible from the Doppler sound.

Pulse oximetry and neonatal ECG are both established methods for determining the heart rate in newborns. However, both have limitations. Any one method may not be ideal, and ECG, oximetry, and Doppler are likely to complement one another in severely compromised neonates. Oximetry requires a significant capillary blood flow, and does not function during the first minute or so after birth even in a healthy neonate. Because it requires a good capillary blood flow, it may not function well in compromised neonates until after resuscitation has been successful. Typically, it takes over a minute after birth for the oximeter to register a heart rate, even in healthy-term neonates. This delay is likely to be significantly longer in compromised neonates, especially when the response to resuscitation is not immediate. A visible oximetry tracing is sometimes available for the resuscitation team, but this requires the attendants to look away from the neonate. ECG can also provide both a visible tracing and digital heart rate, but this requires the attendant to look away from the neonate.

ECG depends on the electrical activity of the heart and, at least in moribund newborns, the possibility of pulseless electrical activity (PEA) needs to be considered. PEA has in fact been identified through the use of colour Doppler flow [14], which is essentially a graphic form of Doppler ultrasound. It could therefore be argued that Doppler ultrasound is actually the gold standard.

4.4. Sterility

Many compromised neonates are delivered by caesarean section, and there is increasing recognition of the importance of resuscitation—when required—with an intact umbilical cord. In healthy neonates, a period of up to three minutes before the cord is clamped is increasingly adopted, and the heart rate needs to be determined during this time [15]. This may require the neonatal resuscitation team to be within or very close to the sterile operating field. It is possible to use a sterile stethoscope to determine the neonatal heart rate in this scenario; however, the application of ECG electrodes or an oximeter presents a significant challenge. Pulse oximetry is in any case unsatisfactory in determining the heart rate during the first minute. However, Doppler ultrasound functions perfectly through polythene as a sterile cover, allowing the Doppler sound to be heard and the displayed heart rate to be seen by the team, and without any special adaption of the current equipment.

4.5. Future Development

A major advantage of ECG and oximetry is that they are hands-free after initial application. The possibility of a hands-free precordial Doppler system has been explored recently. A lightweight transducer that is connected to the Doppler machine by a soft, flexible wire makes the system hands-free. It will sit on the neonate's chest as a result of the surface tension of the ultrasound gel alone, remaining in place even with some movement of the neonate [16]. If auscultation for the entry of air to the lungs or observation of the chest is required, the transducer can simply be lifted off, and later reapplied with a little more ultrasound gel.

5. Conclusions

The use of foetal Doppler to determine the neonatal heart rate at birth has recently been explored. Data are limited, but what evidence there is shows that it has the potential for a more accurate and quicker acquisition of the heart rate immediately after birth. Modifications could make the approach more user-friendly, and it is an established low-cost technology.

Funding: There was no external funding, and all work was funded by the author. The review was carried out as the initial part of the author's MPhil (Medical Engineering) thesis.

Acknowledgments: I am grateful to Reza Saatchi for his critical review of the paper.

Conflicts of Interest: I am developing a hands-free Doppler ultrasound transducer as part of my MPhil (Medical Engineering) thesis.

References

1. Wyllie, J.; Perlman, J.M.; Kattwinkel, J.; Wyckoff, M.H.; Aziz, K.; Guinsburg, R.; Kim, H.-S.; Liley, H.; Mildenhall, L.; Simon, W.M.; et al. Part 7: Neonatal Resuscitation. 2015 International Consensus on Cardiopulmonary Resuscitation and Emergency Cardiovascular Care Science with Treatment Recommendations. *Resuscitation* **2015**, *95*, e169–e201. [CrossRef] [PubMed]
2. Kevat, A.C.; Bullen, D.V.R.; David, P.G.; Kamlin, C.O.F. A systematic review of novel technology for monitoring infants and newborn heart rate. *Acta Paediatr.* **2017**, *106*, 710–720. [CrossRef]
3. Zanardo, V.; Parotto, M. Ultrasonic Pocket Doppler, novel technology for fetal and neonatal heart rate assessment. *Resuscitation* **2019**, *145*, 91–92. [CrossRef] [PubMed]
4. Shimabukuro, R.; Takase, K.; Ohde, S.; Kusakawa, I. Handheld fetal Doppler device for assessing heart rate in neonatal resuscitation. *Pediatr. Int.* **2017**, *59*, 1069–1073. [CrossRef] [PubMed]
5. Agrawal, G.; Kumar, A.; Wazir, S.; Kumar, N.C.; Shah, P.; Nigade, A.; Nagar, N.; Kumar, S.; Kumar, K. A comparative evaluation of portable Doppler ultrasound versus electrocardiogram in heart-rate accuracy and acquisition time immediately after delivery: A multicenter observational study. *J. Matern. Fetal Neonatal Med.* **2021**, *34*, 2053–2060. [CrossRef] [PubMed]
6. Goenka, S.; Khan, M.; Koppel, R.I.; Heiman, H.S. Precordial doppler ultrasound achieves earlier and more accurate newborn heart rates in the delivery room. In Proceedings of the 2013 American Academy of Pediatrics National Conference and Exhibition, Orlando, FL, USA, 26–29 October 2013.
7. Kayama, K.; Hosono, S.; Yoshikawa, K.; Kato, R.; Seimiya, A.; Fuwa, K.; Hijikata, M.; Aoki, R.; Okahashi, A.; Nagano, N.; et al. Heart-rate evaluation using fetal ultrasonic Doppler during neonatal resuscitation. *Pediatr. Int.* **2020**, *62*. [CrossRef] [PubMed]
8. Dyson, A.; Jeffrey, M.; Kluckow, M. Measurement of neonatal heart rate using handheld Doppler ultrasound. *Arch. Dis. Child. Fetal Neonatal Ed.* **2016**, *102*, F116–F119. [CrossRef] [PubMed]
9. Lemke, R.P.; Farrah, M.; Byrne, P.J. Use of a new Doppler umbilical cord clamp to measure heart rate in newborn infants in the delivery room. *e-J. Neonatal. Res.* **2011**, *1*, 83–88.
10. Katheria, A.C.; Brown, M.K.; Faksh, A.; Hassen, K.O.; Rich, W.; Lazarus, D.; Steen, J.; Daneshmand, S.S.; Finer, N.N. Delayed Cord Clamping in Newborns Born at Term at Risk for Resuscitation: A Feasibility Randomized Clinical Trial. *J. Pediatr.* **2017**, *187*, 313–317. [CrossRef] [PubMed]
11. Hutchon, D.J.R. Technological developments in neonatal care at birth. *J. Nurs. Care* **2013**, *3*, 218. [CrossRef]
12. Morina, N.; Johnson, P.A.; O'Reilly, M.; Lee, T.-F.; Yaskina, M.; Cheung, P.-Y.; Schmölzer, G.M. Doppler Ultrasound for Heart Rate Assessment in a Porcine Model of Neonatal Asphyxia. *Front. Pediatr.* **2020**, *8*, 18. [CrossRef] [PubMed]
13. Hutchon, D.; Pratesi, S.; Katheria, A. How to Provide Motherside Neonatal Resuscitation with Intact Placental Circulation? *Children* **2021**, *8*, 291. [CrossRef] [PubMed]
14. Van Vonderen, J.J.; Hooper, S.B.; Kroese, J.K.; Roest, A.A.W.; Narayen, I.C.; van Zwet, E.W.; te Pas, A.B. Pulse oximetry measures a lower heart rate at birth compared with electrocardiography. *J. Pediatr.* **2015**, *166*, 49–53. [CrossRef] [PubMed]
15. Concord Neonatal Solution. Available online: https://concordneonatal.com/ (accessed on 5 April 2022).
16. David Hutchon (25 April 2015) Doppler Ultrasound on Manikin Low Res. How to Monitor and Document the Neonatal Heart Rate at Birth. [Video] Doppler Ultrasound on Mankin Low Res—YouTube. Available online: https://www.youtube.com/watch?v=6yBiQxAgvvw (accessed on 5 April 2022).

MDPI

St. Alban-Anlage 66

4052 Basel

Switzerland

Tel. +41 61 683 77 34

Fax +41 61 302 89 18

www.mdpi.com

Children Editorial Office

E-mail: children@mdpi.com

www.mdpi.com/journal/children

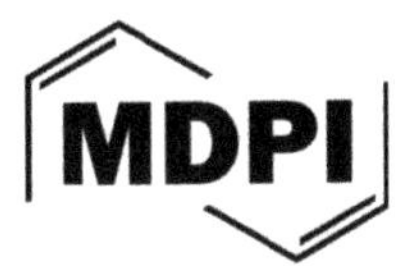